Rheumatology for the House Officer

The First Century 1890-1990
SANS TACHE

Rheumatology for the House Officer

Lourdes C. Corman, M.D.

Associate Professor of Medicine
Department of Medicine
Divisions of General Internal Medicine
and Clinical Immunology, and Rheumatology
University of Florida
Gainesville, Florida

Carolyn L. Bell, M.D.

Associate Professor of Medicine
Department of Medicine
Section of Rheumatology
University of Wisconsin
Madison, Wisconsin

N. Lawrence Edwards, M.D.

Associate Professor of Medicine
Department of Medicine
Division of Clinical Immunology and Rheumatology
University of Florida
Chief, Section of Rheumatology
Veterans Administration Medical Center
Gainesville, Florida

Catherine E. Harmon, M.D.

Associate Professor of Medicine
Department of Medicine
Chief, Division of Rheumatology
Medical College of Ohio
Toledo, Ohio

Illustrated by N. Lawrence Edwards, M.D.

SANS TACHE

WILLIAMS & WILKINS
Baltimore • Hong Kong • London • Sydney

Editor: Michael G. Fisher
Associate Editor: Marjorie Kidd Keating
Copy Editor: Eden Delcher
Designer: Bob Och
Illustration Planner: Lorraine Wrzosek
Production Coordinator: Raymond E. Reter
Cover Designer: Dan Pfisterer

428 East Preston Street
Baltimore, Maryland 21202, USA

Accurate indications, adverse reactions, and dosage schedules for drugs are provided in this book, but it is possible that they may change. The reader is urged to review the package information data of the manufacturers of the medications mentioned.

Printed in the United States of America

Library of Congress Cataloging in Publication Data

Rheumatology for the house officer/Lourdes C. Corman . . . [et al.]; illustrated by N. Lawrence Edwards.
p. cm.
Includes bibliographies and index.
ISBN 0-683-02143-5
1. Rheumatology—Handbooks, manuals, etc. I. Corman, Lourdes C.
[DNLM:1. Rheumatism—diagnosis. 2. Rheumatism—therapy. WE 544 R4722]
RC927.R484 1990
616.7'23—dc20
DNLM/DLC
for Library of Congress 89-16576
CIP
1 2 3 4 5 6 7 8 9 10
90 91 92 93 94

Preface

The four of us are practicing academic rheumatologists and internists with individual areas of interest and two common goals which we hope to achieve with this manual.

Our first goal is to assist you, our readers, in feeling comfortable in the evaluation and treatment of patients with rheumatic complaints. To accomplish this we will share with you our approach to these patients and our collection of "pearls" acquired over the years from teachers, patients, and each other. This manual is clearly not an exhaustive treatise of all there is to know in rheumatology—there are excellent textbooks, monographs, and journal articles to accomplish such a task. Rather, it should teach you enough that you will know what specific diagnoses you need to pursue with further reading for the benefit of your patient. At the end of each chapter, we have provided a few references if you seek greater detail.

Our second goal in writing this manual is to let you share in the enjoyment we derive from the practice of rheumatology. Rheumatic diseases are an internist's dream in that only by maintaining interest and expertise in general internal medicine can we provide optimal care for our patients. As a subspecialty, rheumatology satisfies our scientific curiosity by keeping us abreast of ongoing discoveries in the areas of molecular biology, intermediary metabolism, immunology, pharmacology, and other basic sciences. Treatment of patients with rheumatic complaints is a challenge to our creativity. A tailor-made therapeutic approach to any given patient takes into account the drugs available, the patient's physiologic reserve, the expected clinical course of the illness, and the patient's own economic and social situation. Finally on a personal "doctoring" level, there is little that is more rewarding than seeing a patient ravaged by rheumatoid arthritis, or incapacitated by chronic low back pain, or on death's door from a systemic vasculitis, improve and get back to normal function.

This manual is organized in four parts. The first part comprises the approach to the diagnosis of rheumatic disease. It includes definitions, as well as overviews of the history and physical findings, the use of laboratory and radiologic tests, and the principles of clinical epidemiology that help us to interpret the findings. We suggest that you read this section as a unit and then move on to Part II which covers the regional pain syndromes. In Part III we highlight specific diseases, and in Part IV, we cover therapeutic approaches and how to assess their efficacy.

We look forward to hearing from you with any suggestions you may have about how we can improve this manual the next time around. Please note that we intersperse he/him/his with she/her/hers throughout the book. We hope this keeps us from offending anyone.

Lourdes C. Corman, M.D.
Carolyn L. Bell, M.D.
N. Lawrence Edwards, M.D.
Catherine E. Harmon, M.D.

Acknowledgments

We wish to thank Nancy Collins, editor at Williams & Wilkins, for bringing this project to our attention, and Margie Keating for her continuous support and encouragement. Many of our colleagues have generously shared their expertise with us by critically reading several chapters. We are grateful to Dr. Brad Bender, Dr. George Caranasos, Dr. Richard Davidson, Dr. Peter Gearen, Dr. Frank Graziano, Dr. Rodger Israel, and Dr. John Meuleman, for their contributions. Finally, thanks to our families for their encouragement, and to our typists, Kaye Battell and Loreen Eschliman.

Contents

PART IV

Overview of Treatment of Rheumatic Diseases

PART I.

TOOLS IN THE DIAGNOSIS OF RHEUMATIC DISEASES

Chapter 1

Important Definitions

The diagnosis and treatment of rheumatic diseases are based on the recognition of patterns of affected joints and other organ involvement, and confirmation of our clinical diagnosis by serologic, hematologic, radiographic, and pathologic findings. Certain terms are used so often in rheumatology that it is important to begin any manual like this one with some definitions.

ADL activities of daily living.

**ARA* American Rheumatism Association, an organization, now over 50 years old, established for the purpose of shedding some light into the classification, diagnosis, and treatment of rheumatic disease and for encouraging research into disease pathogenesis. The ARA has been responsible for the development of testable *CRITERIA* used in the diagnosis of many rheumatic diseases.

**ARA* Criteria are lists of symptoms, signs, and other objective findings that can be used in combination to diagnose or classify a rheumatic syndrome. Criteria have been developed by select members of the ARA for the diagnoses of rheumatoid arthritis, systemic lupus erythematosus, acute gouty arthritis, systemic sclerosis, Reiter's syndrome, ankylosing spondylitis, and juvenile rheumatoid arthritis. Most of these criteria have been tested for sensitivity and specificity in populations of patients with the disorder and appropriate control patients. The ARA criteria perform *better* as a diagnostic test than almost any isolated laboratory or radiologic diagnostic test available.

arthralgia pain in the joints.

*Please note that the ARA has recently changed its name to the American College of Rheumatology (ACR).

arthritis inflammation of a joint(s) as manifested by the cardinal signs of rubor, dolor, calor, and tumor (redness, pain, heat, and swelling).

articular cartilage a specialized cartilage (hyaline) that covers the surface of the two or more bones that face the joint space. In synovial joints, the joint capsule is lined by synovial membrane. The articular cartilage is not covered by synovium normally. It merges with the joint capsule synovial membrane at its periphery.

autoimmunity refers to the presence of a humoral or cellular immune response to self antigens. Many systemic rheumatic diseases are characterized by autoimmunity.

bursa is a closed sac lined with synovium-like tissue and filled with synovial fluid. Bursae occur normally over bony prominences and between myofascial planes subject to friction, for example, over the patella and the greater trochanter. Approximately 100 distinct bursae have been identified. They may occasionally communicate freely with the synovial or joint cavity and its fluid.

bursitis inflammation and pain of a bursa.

Clinical Rheumatology covers a vast array of clinical syndromes from the well out-patient with a regional pain disorder to the intensive care unit moribund patient with multiple organ failure.

dermatomal distribution of pain follows the area of skin supplied by a single afferent nerve fiber from a single dorsal root. These have been mapped out for the entire body, and although they tend to overlap considerably, they usually allow you to localize the spinal level fairly well by noting the area of the body affected.

enthesopathy inflammation at the enthesis.

enthesis the site where tendons or ligaments attach to bone and which is characteristically involved in the group of rheumatic diseases known as the seronegative spondyarthritides.

entrapment syndromes neuropathies seen secondary to pressure on a nerve or its vascular supply by other tissues, usually musculotendinous structures. For example, carpal tunnel syndrome due to compression of the median nerve in the carpal tunnel.

joints the connections between two separate skeletal structures. There are several types of joints. The two types most likely to be affected by rheumatic disease are the diarthrodial or synovial joints, and the fibrous or cartilaginous joints.

joint capsule the enclosure of ligaments and fibrous tissue that surround the joint. It attaches to the distal and proximal perimetry of bony structures (and/or articular cartilage) that face each other in the joint.

kyphosis an abnormal curvature of the spine with the convexity pointed posteriorly due to destruction of the affected vertebra, same as "hump back" or hunch-back.

kyphoscoliosis kyphosis combined with scoliosis.

lordosis an antero-posterior curvature of the spine with the convexity pointed anteriorly. There is normally a small degree of lordosis in the cervical and lumbar areas of the spine.

lordoscoliosis lordosis combined with scoliosis.

meniscal cartilage an intra-articular fibrocartilage of the knee.

muscle insertion the more movable point of attachment of a muscle.

muscle origin is the less movable of the two points of attachment of a muscle. It is usually located more proximal than the insertion.

myalgia painful muscles.

myofascial pain pain in the muscle and perimuscular structures that is often accompanied by the presence of trigger points and tender points in the muscle.

myopathy any abnormality or disease of the muscles.

neuralgia pain of a severe, throbbing, or stabbing quality that occurs in the distribution of a nerve and is due to injury or involvement of a nerve in the syndrome.

neuropathy a disease of the peripheral nervous system. It may involve sensory and motor nerves at their most distal distribution producing a stocking-glove polyneuropathy, or one single nerve producing neuritis.

orthotics the use of orthopedic appliances to improve joint well-being and function.

osteopenia a decrease in the bone mass noted by radiography. Osteopenia is a common finding in osteomalacia, osteoporosis, and other metabolic bone diseases. (See Chapter 38.)

osteophytes bony outgrowths from an existing bony structure. When present in the vertebrae, they are horizontally oriented.

palindromic relapsing or recurring with symptom-free intervals.

pannus the exhuberant growth of synovium that invades into the joint and over the articular surface in rheumatoid arthritis, and other inflammatory arthritides.

periosteitis inflammation of the fibrous membrane (periosteum) that covers the surface of a bone.

plexitis disease involving a nerve plexus, e.g., brachial or sciatic plexopathy.

psychogenic conditions with a mental or emotional origin or causation.

referred pain pain which does not originate from the areas of the body where it is felt. It includes pain from internal organs that may present as a regional pain syndrome (e.g., angina pain presenting as elbow, shoulder or neck pain), or the pattern of pain distribution from a joint, bursa, or tendon to more remote areas (e.g., knee pain from disease of the hip).

rheumatology the study of rheumatic disease. The word is derived from the Greek *reuma* meaning flow or flux, and *rheum*, a mucous or watery discharge.

Rheumatic diseases any local or systemic disorder that presents with symptoms or signs related to the joints and/or the rest of the musculoskeletal system. Terms used in the past include "collagen vascular" and "connective tissue" diseases.

ROM range of motion of a joint. The normal ROM for each joint in any given plane is specific for that joint and depends on the anatomy and health of the joint. It can be assessed *passively* with the examiner producing the motion, or observed during *active* motion where the patient initiates and concludes all movements.

sclerotomal pain pain that is felt in the distribution of the primitive somatic segment.

scoliosis a lateral curvature of the spine.

spondyarthropathies (or spondyloarthropathies) are a group of arthritides that involve the axial skeleton and sometimes the peripheral joints, characterized by absence of rheumatoid factor in the patient's serum (seronegative).

seropositive (as opposed to seronegative) refers to the presence in serum of rheumatoid factor, an antibody (usually of the IgM class) with specificity for the class specific end of the IgG molecule (also known as the Fc fragment).

soft tissue rheumatism, also known as *non-articular rheumatism,* comprises all musculoskeletal complaints that involve non-bony, non-articular tissues. For example, muscles, tendons, bursae, ligaments, and neurovascular structures.

syndesmophytes a bony outgrowth due to ossification of the outer fibers of the annulus fibrosus of the intervertebral discs. They have a vertical orientation.

synovium the tissue lining the joint capsule that normally ends at the periphery of the articular cartilage without extending into the joint space.

tender points painful areas within a muscle that are sometimes indurated. They occur typically in fibromyalgia/fibrositis.

tendonitis is inflammation of a tendon sheath.

tenosynovitis inflammation of a tendon sheath and surrounding synovium.

TENS Transcutaneous Electrical Nerve Stimulator (see Chapter 47).

trigger points discrete myofascial areas that on palpation produce pain at a distance from it.

trigger finger or snapping finger seen in association with tenosynovitis of the flexor tendor sheaths and associated nodular enlargement of the tendon and stenosis of the sheath. During flexion, the affected finger may "lock," producing pain.

weakness loss of muscle power or strength. May be generalized or localized, neuropathic, myopathic, central, or psychogenic.

SUGGESTED READINGS

1. *Dictionary of the Rheumatic Diseases.* Volume I: Signs and Symptoms—prepared by ARA Glossary Committee, American Rheumatism Association. New York: Contact Associates International Ltd., 1985.

2. *Dictionary of the Rheumatic Diseases.* Volume II: Diagnostic Testing—prepared by ARA Glossary Committee, American Rheumatism Association. New York: Contact Associates International Ltd., 1985.

3. *Stedman's Medical Dictionary,* 23rd edition, Baltimore; Williams and Wilkins, 1982.

Chapter 2

Clues for Diagnosis —The History

The rheumatic diseases comprise more than a hundred well-recognized clinical syndromes with multiple combinations of symptoms and physical findings that range from widespread vasculitis to localized bursitis. Making the correct diagnosis of an illness has been likened to constructing a map, or filling in a picture, that leads us to the correct diagnosis by pattern recognition. The particulars of each map or picture are filled in from details of the clinical history and confirmed by the physical findings and selected diagnostic tests. As the illness progresses, the history alone may be sufficient to complete the map. In fact, one reason the consultant seeing the patient well into her illness may seem quite astute is that, by the time the consultant is called in, the illness may have evolved sufficiently that a recognizable pattern has developed.

A. IMPORTANCE OF THE CLINICAL HISTORY

In rheumatology, a complete history covering the present illness, past medical history, family history, and review of systems is a must. Examples that illustrate the importance of a complete history abound. A patient may present with an acute polyarthritis due to an allergic serum sickness reaction from the antibiotic prescribed for a urinary tract infection. A severely deformed but minimally painful ankle or knee may be due to diabetic neuropathy and associated Charcot joint. The acutely inflamed tenosynovitis of a young man may be due to gonococcal arthritis or be a harbinger of relapsing leukemia. Pleuritic chest pain, cough, and polyarthralgias may represent pneumococcal pneumonia or drug-induced lupus erythematosus in a setting of cardiac arrhythmias treated with procainamide or quinidine. A recent febrile exanthem in her children or in her classroom may explain the acute arthritis of a teacher with human Parvovirus infection or rheumatic fever. Recent onset of right wrist pain in a weekend gardener may be easily explained once a history of shelling hundreds of peas the previous weekend is obtained.

There is no such thing as useless parts of the history in the rheumatic interview. Both the presence or absence of many symptoms and illnesses contribute to the diagnostic exercise. In addition, while obtaining the clinical history, other purposes of the medical interview are being accomplished. You are beginning to observe the patient's demeanor, movements, and limitations and are getting to know him. The patient, in turn, is beginning to establish a relationship with you.

This process of establishing trust during the initial interview has been described as the *''therapeutic content''* of the interview. To the extent possible, you and the patient should both be comfortable. This assures that both of you will be willing to take the time necessary to at least sketch out your diagnostic map. Finally, never assume that you and the patient give the same meaning to certain words. For example, asking a patient if there has been fever may elicit a yes which you may interpret as a documented elevation in body temperature, while the patient may in fact be describing recent fever blisters.

Beware of the tendency to evaluate pain and disease as either "real" or "in the patient's mind." This dichotomized model of illness is inaccurate, unfair to the patient, and destructive to your diagnostic and therapeutic efforts. All pain and illness is real, since pain and illness are experienced at the cortical level.

B. SPECIFICS IN THE HISTORY

There are five elements of the history that must be elicited in *every* patient being evaluated for a rheumatic disease.

1. *Why is the patient here and now?* In other words, what are the chief complaint and the history of present illness. Additional questions that help further delineate the illness are an obvious corollary. Questions like: Did you ever have this before? When and how long? What makes it better? What makes it worse? If there is pain, does it appear to be related to motion of the area or unrelated to it? Is it articular? If so, is the patient describing *arthri-*

tis (with inflammation and pain) or *arthralgia* (with pain only)? If the patient complains of arthritis, ask if at the time of the symptoms anyone looking at the patient would have been able to notice it, suggesting swelling and redness and therefore active synovitis. *How many joints* have been involved and in what pattern? Has there been overuse as might occur in an athlete, an artist, or with certain occupations? If the illness has a recurrent pattern, establishing when the last episode occurred and concentrating on it while it is fresh in the patient's mind will often be helpful. Any *systemic symptoms* like fever, malaise, weight loss, or any trauma preceding it? Any *other organ involvement* like diarrhea, urethritis, or some other preceding infection? Any other symptoms or signs temporarily related to this illness like rashes, skin tightening, chest pain, mouth ulcers, weakness, etc.? Any *recent immunizations, drugs,* or similar illness in their home, work, or school environment? Any *family history* of arthritis, if so what did the relative look like? Was there obvious deformity of the joints or skeleton? If you find that the patient appears unable to describe a chief complaint, but rather rambles on about unsatisfactory treatment from other doctors, you are eliciting a very important clue which some of us call "the absent chief complaint" presentation of somatizers.

2. *What is the patient's usual state of health?* This amount to the past medical history and includes earlier and current illnesses, previous hospitalizations, surgeries, immunizations, and habits that may affect health. This becomes extremely important in filling in the clinical picture so that rheumatic syndromes associated with systemic conditions may become obvious. You should also look into the social situation including how many children at home, sexual preferences and habits, job, level of stress, transportation, etc. This will become very important in planning therapy.
3. What *medications* and *over-the-counter products* (laxatives, aspirin, vitamins, etc.) does the patient take? Include tobacco, alcohol, and illegal drugs. This is extremely important to know so that you may consider (a) if any of these items could be producing the symptoms, or (b) if they might later interfere with necessary therapy. When a patient develops an illness while on any medication, you should *always* consider that the illness may be due

to an adverse or idiosyncratic reaction to the drug. Who knows, you may be the first one to report the association!

4. Has the patient *ever* experienced a bad reaction from a drug or any over-the-counter product? Does the reaction sound like a "real" type I IgE mediated hypersensitivity response or some other adverse effect? If you find that the drug in question would truly be best in the situation, you need to make sure the patient understands why this is necessary and is willing to try the drug again.
5. A fifth question you must ask, especially if the complaint is thought to be due to an injury or accident is: *Is there any litigation or disability determination pending?* A positive answer does not prove or even suggest lack of organicity or psychogenic cause. However, it does help evaluate the likelihood of recovery and the prognosis.

If your interview time is running short, leave the review of systems to the time when you do the screening examination.

Finally, at the end of the interview you should always ask if there are any specific concerns or diagnoses that the patient would like addressed. Not infrequently, friends or relatives have discussed some diagnoses with the patient which they fear may be the cause for the illness. Until these concerns are discussed, the patient may not feel totally at ease with your diagnosis or treatment.

SUGGESTED READINGS

1. Bates B. *A Guide to Physical Examination,* fourth edition. Philadelphia: J. B. Lippincott, Co. 1988.

2. Campbell EJM. The diagnosing mind. Lancet. 1987; 1:849-51.

Chapter 3

Clues for Diagnosis—The Physical Examination

A screening physical examination should be performed in every patient with a rheumatic complaint and supplemented by specific maneuvers when necessary. In subsequent chapters, the anatomy of specific regions will be covered in more detail. This chapter will review important elements in the physical examination relevant to the rheumatic diseases. The examination may be organized and performed by organ system, by regional area, or by a combination of both. Regardless of the approach you prefer, try to keep it methodical lest you forget an area.

THE PHYSICAL EXAMINATION

It actually begins with the medical interview. This is a good time to observe the patient without the distraction of concentrating on eliciting a specific physical finding. When you begin the examination, make sure both you and the patient are as comfortable as possible. In general, be nosy about scars, contractures, lesions, etc. that the patient may have forgotten to tell you about earlier. Deciding whether a finding is or is not abnormal is one of the more difficult judgments you make during the physical examination.

1. *Vital signs and general observations*
   Check the body temperature as you would in any other patient. Rheumatic disease patients often have *fever* as part of the clinical features of their illness. In addition the illness and/or the treatment may increase the risk of infectious complications. Monitoring the *blood pressure* is essential in any patient, but in the rheumatology clinic, it is especially important in patients with scleroderma, lupus,

vasculitis, and mixed connective tissue disease. Hypertensive complications from involvement of the extra- or intra-renal arteries and arterioles often present with little else but increased BP and abnormal urine sediment.

The *respiratory rate* and the *pulse* are non-specific measures of cardiopulmonary function, overall health, and anxiety. On occasion, they may reflect a drug effect.

Observe how the patient stands from the chair, any limitations or abnormality of stance or gait, ability to heel walk towards you and toe walk away from you to detect weakness of the L_5, and S_1 motor roots. Have her stand on one leg, then the other. If there is a history of *weakness*, asking the patient to squat or, if too weak, observing the manner in which the patient stands up from the chair helps determine the degree of limitation. This is later supplemented by having him go up and down a step and by checking proximal limb girdle and neck strength.

With the patient standing with her back to you, check the back for *scoliosis* and pelvic tilt. If the curvature present on standing disappears on bending forward, it was due to pelvic tilt rather than scoliosis. Check for spinal tenderness and mobility in all four planes—forward flexion, backward extension, lateral bending, and rotation. It is also a good point at which to do a Schober test for spinal distraction (see Chapter 16). Measure *occiput to wall* distance in spondylytic patients with their heels against the wall and without bending the neck to follow disease progression. *Tender/trigger points* in the occiput, at the level of C_7, T_7, paraspinal musculature, episacral fat pads, sciatic notches, trochanteric bursae, and fascia latae tendons can be done at this time. The typical bulging of a *Baker's cyst* in the popliteal space can be looked for now, then use this opportunity to complete your examination of the skin of the back.

2. *Skin and extremities* (see also Chapter 41)
This includes the *scalp*, the skin of the trunk (front and back), head, and extremities. To some extent, the *mucous membranes* are part of this examination, but they are examined during the head and neck and genital examinations. The scalp is difficult to examine completely, and this examination can be assisted by asking the patient if there have been any changes in the scalp. Patches of scarring alopecia suggestive of *discoid lupus* of the scalp and "dandruff" or

"seborrhea" that are actually *psoriasis* can be detected. Other preferred areas of involvement by psoriasis include the intergluteal fold, the area behind the ears, and the extensor surfaces of the elbow.

Rashes of any type should be noted, including the classic rash of *erythema multiforme,* the atrophic scars with a red border of *discoid lupus,* the *erythema chronicum migrans* of Lyme disease, the malar rash of systemic lupus, the heliotrope-hued periorbital edema of *dermatomyositis,* the redundancy and hyperelasticity of some of the true collagen diseases, and the vesicular painful rash of *herpes zoster* in a dermatomal distribution. The extremities may show the painful, warm, discolored swelling of fasciitis due to *erythema nodosum,* ulcerations over the distal tibia seen in *rheumatoid vasculitis,* the classic necrotizing deep lesion of *pyoderma gangrenosum,* or the non-specific maculopapular eruption of drug hypersensitivity. Look for *petechiae* associated with thrombocytopenia or vasculitis. Bullous lesions and hypertrichosis of sun-exposed areas suggest *porphyria. Nodules* may be due to tophi, xanthomas, ganglia, rheumatic fever, or malignancy (including the pigmented, non-tender nodules of *Kaposi's sarcoma* seen in AIDS patients). Symmetrical nodules associated with hypesthesia suggest *leprosy.* Flat nodules on the skin around the eyes suggest *sarcoidosis.* A petechial/purpuric/ecchymotic rash mostly in the lower extremities suggests *Henoch Schönlein purpura* or *idiopathic thrombocytopenic purpura.* Asymmetric, non-pitting, brawny edema of a distal extremity is seen in reflex neurodystrophy.

This is a good time to look for the telangiectasiae of *CREST* syndrome, primarily in the hands and face, the changes of sclerodactyly, and proximal *scleroderma* with tight bound-down skin. Liver spiders of the upper thorax and linear streaking from scratching reachable areas suggest itching and liver disease and may be due to *primary biliary cirrhosis.* Long fingers (*arachnodactyly*) are seen in *Marfan's* syndrome. Note the presence of *acne,* which, when severe, may be associated with an arthropathy. *Cushing's syndrome* (usually iatrogenic in this population) has telltale signs consisting of increased facial hair, buffalo hump, moon facies, increased supraclavicular fat pads, pigmented striae, truncal obesity, purpuric areas from increased capillary fragility.

The *nails* and *nail beds* may show *clubbing* in association with hypertrophic pulmonary osteoarthropathy. Splinter hemorrhages are usually from manual labor, but may also be seen in *bacterial endocarditis*. Horizontal ridges of illness (*Beau's* lines) or arsenic poisoning (*Mees'* lines) occur. The *periungual capillaries,* which are not normally obvious to the naked eye, may become dilated and tortuous and easily noted in scleroderma, lupus, or dermatomyositis. Look for *stellate stars;* they are healed counterparts of small ulcerations of the fingertips seen in scleroderma and related overlap syndromes. Look for transient color changes in the hands and feet seen in *Raynaud's* phenomenon. Small painful "splinter-like" lesions in the extremities (not just the nail beds) should be thought due to a *septic vasculitis* until proven otherwise by negative blood cultures. *Dactylitis* of a toe leading to a *''sausage'' toe* may be seen in Reiter's syndrome.

3. *Head, neck, ears, and nose*
   In addition to examining the scalp as previously mentioned, check the *temporal arteries* for tenderness and pulsations. Examine the *temporo-mandibular joint* and the range of motion of the neck. Press the frontal, ethmoid, and maxillary *sinus* areas to elicit tenderness. The external ear may show evidence of deformity of the helix following an episode of redness, warmth, and pain suggestive of *relapsing polychondritis* (RP). A similar process in the bridge of the nose may represent RP or *Wegener's granulomatosis.* Look at the nasal mucosa. Identify ulcerations, *polyps* (which may be associated with hypersensitivity to aspirin and other non-steroidals), discharge, dryness. Look for enlargement of the *lacrimal* or *parotid glands* (see Chapter 31).

   In the neck, check the *thyroid* and the carotid pulsations. Palpate the sternocleidomastoid muscle for tenderness. When the patient is supine, look for neck vein distention and hepatojugular reflux characteristic of *heart failure.* In a patient with shortness of breath, listen over the trachea for stridor. *Laryngeal obstruction* secondary to tracheal inflammation and collapse can be seen in Wegnener's granulomatosis and relapsing polychondritis.
4. *Eyes* (see also Chapter 42)
   The *conjunctivae* may be infected. There may be *corneal* ulcerations from a sicca syndrome. The pupil may be irregular from previous *iritis/uveitis* and synechiae. A bluish tinge to the sclera is seen in *osteogenesis imperfecta* and perforation of the sclera (*scleromalacia perforans*) may occur in rheumatoid arthritis. *Dislocated lens* suggests

Marfan's syndrome or homocystinuria. *Optic atrophy* and retinal hemorrhages may occur from vasculitis. "Cotton-wool" exudates (*cytoid bodies*) in the retina are seen in lupus. Behçet's syndrome and ankylosing spondylitis also commonly affect the uveal tract and conjunctiva.

5. *Mouth*
   Characteristic inability to open the mouth from lip border to lip border to 4 cm or more is seen in scleroderma, and can be measured to follow disease progression. Look for *absent pool of saliva* under the tongue in xerostomia. *Ulcers of the oral mucosa* may be painful (aphthous ulcer or canker sore) suggestive of Behçet's syndrome, or asymptomatic as in Reiter's syndrome. A high-arched palate is seen in Marfan's syndrome.
6. *Lymph nodes*
   Check the head and neck, axillae, epitrochlear, inguinal, and popliteal areas for adenopathy. Small, less than 1 cm., soft, minimally painful nodes are often seen in many rheumatic diseases. Anything larger or harder should raise the possibility of a malignancy.
7. *Chest and breasts*
   Listen and percuss the anterior, posterior, and lateral thorax to evaluate the lungs. You're looking for evidence of a *pleural effusion* (dull percussion and decreased breath sounds) that may be seen with rheumatoid arthritis, lupus, scleroderma, etc. Late inspiratory rales that don't clear with coughing may be due to *heart failure.* "Velcro"-like rales of *pulmonary fibrosis* can occur in scleroderma, mixed connective tissue disease, rheumatoid arthritis, Sjögren's syndrome, polymyositis, lupus, etc. In women, careful inspection of the breasts is indicated.
8. *Heart and pulses*
   Increased P2 and right parasternal lift from *right ventricular hypertrophy* is seen with pulmonary hypertension that may develop in scleroderma and mixed connective tissue disease. The high-pitched early diastolic blow of *aortic insufficiency* best heard at Erb's point (3rd left intercostal space) with the patient leaning forward in full expiration should be sought in patients with ankylosing spondylitis. *Mitral valve prolapse* with its characteristic mid-systolic click and murmur best heard at the apex is associated with fibromyalgia.

   Arterial pulses of the arms may be absent in Takayasu's arteritis and in temporal arteritis. These may be examined during the musculoskeletal examination and/or during the examination of the extremities.

9. *Abdominal, rectal, and genital areas*
Bruits from arteritis of the abdominal arteries may be heard in polyarteritis nodosa. Other findings may be noted, such as pain on palpation of the *epigastrium* from the use of non-steroidal anti-inflammatory drugs, a right lower quadrant mass in *Crohn's disease,* or *ascites* in lupus patients with serositis. *Hemoccult positive stools* due to anti-inflammatories or from vasculitis and bowel ischemia may occur. Genital ulceration and unrecognized *balanitis* may be seen in patients with Reiter's syndrome, although asymptomatic genital ulcers in females may also occur in Behçet's syndrome.
10. *Musculoskeletal and neurovascular*
The regional specific maneuvers and neurovascular findings are reviewed in Chapters 11-19 on the regional pain syndromes. For each joint, establish the active *range of motion* and any tenderness localized to specific structures. The range of motion is best measured by a goniometer. Look for evidence of tenosynovitis—swelling and warmth of tendons and joints, effusions, and limitation of motion. Tender, "fleshy," apparently thickened MCPs may be an early manifestation of polyarthritis or the result of heavy manual labor.

    Abnormalities in joint and bone alignment and deviations should be noted. *Weakness* of proximal and distal musculature and, when necessary, specific muscle groups is tested by impeding normal motion. The usual grading scale is 0 to 5. No motion is 0, and grade 5 normal strength. Grade 4 is full motion against gravity and some resistance, grade 3 is motion against gravity only, grade 2 with gravity eliminated, and grade 1 minimal muscle contractibility without motion. If you want to measure *grip strength,* inflate a BP cuff to 20 mm and ask the patient to squeeze with each hand. Proximal weakness is more commonly associated with myopathy, distal weakness with neuropathy. Involvement of specific nerves in an asymmetric fashion suggests *mononeuritis multiplex* and underlying vasculitis (although diabetes mellitus is also a recognized etiology). Bell's palsy is usually idiopathic but may be due to Lyme disease, scleroderma, or an overlap syndrome.

    Look for symmetric and proportioned muscle bulk. Evaluate joint laxity from *benign hypermobility* or a connective tissue disease by passive opposition of the thumbs to the distal forearm, hyperextension of the fingers, elbows and heels, and hyperflexion of the ankles. Ulnar deviation of the fingers from joint laxity is characteristic of *Jaccoud's arthropathy* seen after rheumatic fever with heart involvement or secondary to lupus erythematosus.

Elicit the *deep tendon reflexes*, abnormal reflexes, and sensory and proprioceptive functions. When there is dermatomal pain, the following list is helpful in localizing the nerve root.

Dermatome levels

C_2	= top of head
C_4, C_5	= anterior and posterior neck
C_6	= shoulder and thumb
C_8	= 4th and 5th fingers and elbow
T_5, T_6	= episgastrium
T_{10}	= umbilicus
L_1	= groin
L_4	= in-step and big toe
L_5	= anterior shin, bottom of the foot and 2-4 toes
S_1	= little toe and lateral malleolus
S_2	= posterior calf, heel and buttock
S_3, S_4, S_5, and C_1	= perianal area.

SUGGESTED READINGS

1. Polley HF, Hunder GG. *Rheumatologic Interviewing and Physical Examination of the Joints*, second edition, Philadelphia: W. B. Saunders Company, 1978.

2. Bates B. *A Guide to Physical Examination*, fourth edition. Philadelphia: J. B. Lippincott Co. 1988.

Chapter 4

Help from the Laboratory—Hemogram, Chemistry Profile, and Urinalysis

The routine hematology and chemistry laboratories can be helpful in the evaluation and diagnosis of rheumatic illnesses, and are part of the necessary monitoring for toxicity of antirheumatic therapies.

A. COMPLETE BLOOD COUNT, DIFFERENTIAL, AND PLATELET COUNT

I. *The red blood cells.* Many patients with chronic rheumatic diseases are anemic. The *anemia* is usually normochromic and normocytic, the so-called "anemia of chronic disease." This is frequently seen with rheumatoid arthritis. The serum iron, transferrin, and total iron-binding capacity are often low or normal, and the reticulocyte count is often inappropriately low. Patients with chronic arthritis on non-steroidal drugs may also be anemic from iron deficiency associated with gastrointestinal blood loss from mucosal damage (gastritis or peptic ulceration). These patients may have hypochromic, normocytic cells, but iron studies are not typical for iron deficiency because of the underlying anemia of chronic disease. If the red cell indices suggest macrocytosis or the polymorphonuclear leukocytes show hypersegmentation, levels of folate and cobalamin should be obtained. In patients with systemic lupus, a Coombs' positive *hemolytic anemia* may occur. In these patients, the direct Coombs' test looking for antibody-coated red cells is positive. The peripheral smear will show evidence of hemolysis. In contrast, a positive indirect Coombs' test is usually of little clinical consequence.

II. The *white cell count* in most rheumatic syndromes is normal but may be high or low. The differential is of little help as a diagnostic test, but is helpful in monitoring toxicity of various antirheumatic drugs. *Felty's syndrome* (a variant of rheumatoid arthritis) is characterized by leukopenia and splenomegaly. SLE is often associated with leukopenia and lymphopenia, while many of the vasculitides are associated with leukocytosis.

III. The *platelet count* is usually elevated in inflammatory conditions because it acts as an acute phase reactant. Lupus and some medications may have an associated thrombocytopenia. Most patients with an acute rheumatic illness have thrombocytosis which is only rarely over 800,000. When the level approaches 1×10^6, a myeloproliferative syndrome is more likely.

B. CHEMISTRY PROFILE AND URINE ANALYSIS

Frequently used serum chemistries include the serum creatinine and electrolytes, glucose, calcium, phosphorus, alkaline phosphatase, uric acid, albumin, bilirubin, and transaminases. The serum *creatinine* and the routine urinalysis are of greatest help in assessing renal function in patients with lupus or vasculitis or who are on drugs with potential nephrotoxicity like gold, D-penicillamine, nonsteroidals, and cyclophosphamide. The glomerular filtration rate is measured with a 24° urine collection for creatinine and a simultaneous serum creatinine. The total amount of daily *proteinuria* can also be quantitated in this collection. The presence of red cells and casts, especially red cell casts, in a urinalysis is the most sensitive indicator of *acute nephritis* even in the absence of an elevated creatinine. The presence of eosinophils in the urine should suggest a drug-related interstitial nephritis.

Elevated levels of *alkaline phosphatase* suggests either liver or bone disease. Paget's disease of bone, vitamin D deficiency (with associated osteomalacia or rickets), healing fractures, hyperparathyroidism, and metastatic bone disease can all be associated with increased levels of this enzyme. Any liver disease with obstruction of the biliary system can also produce an increased level.

Multiple drugs may first manifest impending toxicity by producing elevation of *liver enzymes*. Elevated transaminases are suggestive of hepatocellular damage and should suggest to you that the patient's illness is involving the liver, that your therapy is damaging this organ (for example, aspirin, other non-steroidal anti-inflammatory drugs, methotrexate, allopurinol, etc.), or that there is primary disease of the liver (e.g., viral hepatitis).

C. COAGULATION STUDIES
A prolonged activated partial thromboplastin time (PTT) should make you think of a congenital or acquired coagulopathy. When seen in a patient with a hypercoagulable state without a bleeding diathesis, a "lupus anti-coagulant" is the most likely cause. This is an antibody directed against phospholipid and is more commonly associated with thrombosis and fetal wastage than with bleeding or lupus (see Chapters 5 and 27).

D. OTHER STUDIES
Stool hemoccult can detect early toxicity from non-steroidals. It is also positive in ischemia of the bowel that may complicate the necrotizing vasculitides.

SUGGESTED READING

1. Wallach J. *Interpretation of diagnostic tests—a handbook synopsis of laboratory medicine,* 4th edition. Boston: Little, Brown, and Co. 1986.

Chapter 5

Help from the Immunology Laboratory: Serology of the Inflammatory Response and Other Rheumatic Serology

Whenever an inflammatory process develops, within minutes to hours from this insult, changes take place in the circulating elements of blood and serum. Since the 1920s, when Westergren first described changes in the rapidity of sedimentation of red blood cells in the serum of pregnant women, physicians have taken advantage of these changes to help diagnose the illness and follow its activity.

ACUTE PHASE REACTANTS

Acute phase reactants are proteins of hepatic origin whose plasma concentrations increase in response to either acute tissue injury or an inflammatory stimulus that releases *interleukin-1* from phagocytic cells. Increases in production of specific and non-specific antibodies by lymphocytes and plasma cells also occur. The individual reactants may be individually measured or their effect measured collectively by means of the erythrocyte sedimentation rate. Acute phase reactants include such coagulation proteins as fibrinogen, prothrombin, Factor VIII and plasminogen; protease inhibitors such as alpha-1-antitrypsin, alpha-1-anti-chymotrypsin and alpha-2-macroglobulin; transport proteins such as haptoglobin, hemopexin, ferritin, and ceruloplasmin; and other proteins including C-reactive protein, alpha-1-acid glycoprotein, alpha-2-globulin, serum amyloid A-related protein, alpha-1-lipoprotein, and lipoproteins. In contrast, the levels of some substances markedly decrease during the inflammatory response, these are called "negative" acute phase reactants and include albumin, prealbumin, transferrin, and serum iron.

The *erythrocyte sedimentation rate* (ESR) measures the distance red blood cells fall in a tube of specified dimensions within one hour. A normal ESR is less than or equal to 20 mm/hr. It is a crude and insensitive method to detect inflammation. For example, it may parallel rheumatoid arthritis activity and is usually normal in osteoarthritis patients. On the other hand, in active systemic lupus erythematosus, it is often low despite the aggressive inflammation present. For the most part, two methods have been used for determining the ESR: the *Westergren* and the *Wintrobe* methods. The Westergren technique employs a longer tube and is not limited by the hematocrit or packed red blood cell volume. It is the preferred method to determine the ESR. Erythrocyte sedimentation rates of over 100 mm/hr are associated with polymyalgia rheumatica with or without giant cell arteritis, various systemic vasculitides, infection, plasma cell dyscrasias, neoplasms, very active and aggressive rheumatoid arthritis, and chronic renal failure.

The *C-reactive protein* increases from less than one to several hundred mg per dl. Like the ESR, it may parallel rheumatoid arthritis activity but values may be low or normal in lupus, scleroderma, and poly/dermatomyositis even in the presence of very active disease. It has been suggested by some authors that a high quantitative measure of CRP in lupus identifies significant infection rather than active lupus. Unfortunately, this methodology is not readily available in most laboratories which usually only provide qualitative reports.

RHEUMATOID FACTOR

Rheumatoid factor (RF) is an antibody specifically directed against antigenic determinants on the Fc portion of human or animal IgG. These antibodies may be of the IgM, IgG, IgA, and even IgD or IgE immunoglobulin class. Classically, *rheumatoid factor is IgM directed against IgG*. The traditional laboratory tests for rheumatoid factor determination are the latex agglutination and sheep red cell agglutination. These detect IgM rheumatoid factor but not IgG rheumatoid factor or any of the other similarly described rheumatoid factors. Nearly 80% of patients with rheumatoid arthritis develop classic rheumatoid factor, that is, IgM directed against IgG, within three to six months of ongoing disease activity in a titer of 1:160 or greater. Therefore, 20% of people who satisfy the ARA criteria for the diagnosis of rheumatoid arthritis do not have IgM rheumatoid factor present in their sera. These seronegative rheumatoid arthritis patients may have IgG, IgA, or IgD rheumatoid factors not identified by the latex agglutination test. High titer (19-S) IgM (classic RF) and/or 7-S IgM rheumatoid factor are often found in patients with rheumatoid vasculitis.

Neither the presence nor the absence of rheumatoid factor is sufficient for confirming or excluding a diagnosis of rheumatoid arthritis. As with most connective tissue diseases, rheumatoid arthritis remains a diagnosis made on clinical grounds. Rheumatoid factor may also be seen in other rheumatic as well as non-rheumatic conditions. For example, a third of patients with scleroderma or with systemic lupus erythematosus will demonstrate rheumatoid factor positivity in a titer greater than or equal to 1:160. Some patients with polymyositis and over 90% of patients with Sjögren's syndrome will also be rheumatoid factor positive. In addition, rheumatoid factor can be seen in a variety of non-rheumatic diseases, including viral infection, parasitic infection, chronic active hepatitis, silicosis, subacute bacterial endocarditis, interstitial pulmonary fibrosis, or any disease with an on-going inflammatory response. Finally, in a population over age 65, a third may be rheumatoid factor positive without any associated connective tissue disease.

COMPLEMENT

The complement system consists of a series of interacting serum proteins which are involved in the metabolism and disposal of immune complexes, microorganisms, and altered host cells by promoting and regulating the inflammatory process. The final outcome of activating the complement cascade is deposition of the immune complex in tissue for disposal, or the lysis of bacteria or abnormal host cells. There are two ways to measure complement proteins, functional assays, and quantitative assays. *Total hemolytic complement* (the CH_{50} assay) is a functional assay which measures the interaction of all the complement components in lysing 50% of the target cells. *Specific complement components* can be measured and quantitated by radial immunodiffusion. There are both inherited and acquired disorders of complement.

Inherited deficiencies of the early components of complement (particularly C_2, C_3, and C_4) are associated with some connective tissue diseases, especially systemic lupus erythematosus. Inherited deficiencies of the later components (C_8, C_9) are associated with recurrent neisserial (e.g., meningococcal and gonococcal) infections. An inherited deficiency of C_3 is also associated with recurrent pyogenic infections.

Inherited C_2 deficiency is the most common inherited deficiency associated with lupus. The lupus seen with inherited complement deficiencies is usually milder than the idiopathic form. Common features include discoid lesions and photosensitivity. Uncommon features include CNS involvement and renal disease. Antibodies to double-stranded DNA and positive immunofluorescent skin tests (the deposition of immunoglobulin and/or complement at the dermal-epidermal junction) are not as common in this form as in idiopathic lupus.

The most common reason why people with lupus have *low complement values* is not due to an inherited deficiency of complement but to activation of complement by immune complex deposition with a decrease in CH_{50} levels and an associated decrease in both C_3 and C_4. Decreased serum complement usually correlates with active lupus and particularly with active lupus nephritis. Decreased serum levels of complement have also been reported in 25% of Sjögren's syndrome patients with vasculitis, although in these patients these values may represent "in vitro" rather than "in vivo" activation. Other connective tissue diseases such as drug-induced lupus, rheumatoid arthritis, dermatomyositis, and scleroderma are characterized by normal serum complement levels. Complement deposition may occur in some systemic vasculitides, and low serum complement levels have been reported in cholesterol-embolic disease (from atheromatous plaques) that can mimic vasculitis.

When low, serum complement levels provide an objective parameter with which to follow activity in SLE and some vasculitides. However, as usual in clinical medicine, treatment is aimed at improving the patient, not just the serum value.

AUTOIMMUNE SEROLOGIES

In addition to the erythrocyte sedimentation rate, rheumatoid factor and complement levels, an additional serologic test is most useful in the diagnosis and treatment of rheumatic diseases: the titer, pattern, and specificity of antinuclear antibodies (ANA). In addition, antibodies to intracytoplasmic enzymes of neutrophils have been described that are highly sensitive and specific for active Wegener's granulomatosis.

Antinuclear Antibodies

The first antinuclear antibody responsible for the LE cell phenomenon was described by Hargraves and his associates in the late 1940s. It consists of a polymorphonuclear leukocyte with a cytoplasmic inclusion later found to be an immune complex consisting of deoxyribonucleoprotein (DNP) and antibody to it. Since the time of Hargraves and the description of the LE cell test, there has been an explosion of well-characterized antigen-antibody systems with antibodies directed against a variety of nuclear constituents, as shown in the Table below.

Table 5.1
Well-Defined Nuclear Antigens to Naturally Occurring Antibodies

DNA
- double-stranded (native) DNA
- single-stranded DNA

Histones
- H1, H2A, H2B, H3, H4
- histone complexes

Non-Histone Proteins
- small RNA-protein particles
- Sm
- nRNP (U1 RNP)
- SS-A/Ro
- SS-B/La
- tRNA synthetases
  - JO-1 (histidyl tRNA synthetase)
  - PL-7 (threonyl tRNA synthetase
  - PL-12 (alanyl tRNA synthetase)
- Mi systems: Mi-1, Mi-2
- Scl-70 (topoisomerase I)
- Ku
- RANA
- MA
- PCNA (cyclin)
- centromere (kinetochore)
- NuMA

Nucleolar Components
- PM-1 (PM-Scl)
- RNA polymerase I
- fibrillarin

ANA Terminology

Complicating the understanding of ANAs is the confusion of ANA terminology. For example, nuclear ribonuclear protein has also been described under the alternative names Mo, U1-RNP, or the ENA complex. Also previously described as part of the ENA complex was the Sm antigen. ENA (or extractable nuclear antigen) is an old term based on the solubility of some antigens in saline buffers. It contains Sm and RNP antigens, SS-A (Ro) and SS-B (La), and others. Use of the term "ENA complex" to denote only Sm and RNP antigens is incorrect. Scl-70 was first described as Scl-1. Because the Scl-1 antigen has a molecular weight of approximately 70,000, it was renamed Scl-70 but now even that appears to be a misnomer since Scl-70 has been identified as a topoisomerase enzyme that assists in the coiling and uncoiling of DNA.

When to Order an ANA

This should be done primarily when a connective tissue disease or an autoimmune disease is strongly suspected (see Chapter 9). The presence or absence of an ANA will then help to confirm or negate your clinical impression. The test is usually performed by an indirect immunofluorescent technique and is a good screening test because it detects a wide variety of different antibodies to nuclear antigens. The test is performed by placing a substrate on a microscope slide. The substrates have traditionally been mouse kidney or liver but now many laboratories are using human tissue culture epithelioid cell lines such as Hep-2 or KB cells. These cells have advantages such as large nuclei, prominent nucleoli, and actively dividing cells. The patient's serum is added to the substrate on the slide, and if antibodies to nuclear components are present in the patient's serum, they will bind to the substrate cell layer on the slide. In order to detect the immune complex formed by the serum antibodies and the nuclear antigens, fluorescein tagged anti-human immunoglobulin is added to the slide. If antibodies to nuclear antigens are present, the anti-human immunoglobulin will attach to the ANAs on the slide and exhibit green immunofluorescence under a fluorescent microscope.

ANA technology is not uniform; there is a great deal of interlaboratory variation in the test, and results from one laboratory may not have the same implications and significance as those from another laboratory. Different laboratories may use different substrates, different titers of significance, different detecting agents, different fluorescent microscopes, and different technicians. These variables lead to a great deal of subjectivity and differences in ANA technology. To assist you in interpreting an ANA result, review the Table of caveats below.

Caveats in the Interpretation of a Positive ANA

1. Finding should be from a reliable laboratory
   (a) find out the substrate used for the test
   (b) ask for the titer of "significance." This is usually accepted as that exhibited by less than 5% of normal controls
   (c) reproducibility of the findings
2. Clinical correlation
3. Age of the patient
4. Use of any ANA-inducing drugs
5. Specificity of the ANA

Patterns of Nuclear Immunofluorescence

There are four basic patterns of immunofluorescent ANAs: homogeneous, rim, speckled, and nucleolar. *Homogeneous* or diffuse staining of the nucleus is characteristically produced by antibodies to *histones, double-stranded DNA*, or *deoxyribonucleoprotein*. The *rim* or *peripheral staining* of the nucleus also signifies antibodies to *double-stranded DNA, deoxyribonucleoprotein*, or histones. The *speckled* or particulate staining within the nucleus is the most commonly reported immunofluorescent ANA pattern, and antibodies to Sm, RNP, SS-B, Scl-70, centromere, and a wide variety of as yet uncharacterized antigen-antibody systems demonstrate speckled nuclear staining. It is not unusual to have a serum with a strongly positive speckled ANA and a negative screen for specific ANAs because the antibody-antigen system responsible for the staining has not yet been identified. Nucleolar staining is characteristically seen in such diseases as lupus, scleroderma, Raynaud's phenomenon and Sjögren's syndrome and is currently under intense investigation.

ANA Positivity in Rheumatic Diseases

Systemic lupus erythematosus is almost always an ANA positive disease with 95-100% of people with *active* systemic lupus ANA positive, so if the ANA is negative in a patient suspected of having SLE, three possibilities should be considered: (1) this is not lupus; (2) the patient has the rare but real condition known as "ANA negative" or "ANA-substrate-dependent lupus," that is, criteria for a diagnosis of lupus are present but the ANA is negative; or (3) lab error.

Rheumatoid arthritis has a 40-60% ANA positivity. ANA positivity usually occurs later in the course of rheumatoid arthritis. In *progressive systemic sclerosis* or scleroderma, 60% of patients are positive on mouse kidney substrate and 90-95% are positive on Hep-2 cells. The reason for the substrate discrepancy is due to the fact that Hep-2 cell substrates are much more likely to detect nucleolar and centromere staining which are quite characteristic of patients with progressive systemic sclerosis. In idiopathic *dermato-polymyositis*, 50% of patients are positive on mouse kidney and 75% of patients are ANA positive on Hep-2 cell substrates. Therefore, despite earlier suggestions that dermato-polymyositis was not an ANA positive disease, with more sensitive technology, a significant portion of idiopathic dermato-polymyositis patients are ANA positive. In *mixed connective tissue disease*, 100% of patients should be ANA positive because 100% of patients with mixed connective tissue disease are positive for antibodies to nuclear ribonuclear protein, which can always be detected by a screening ANA test. *Drug-induced* lupus patients should also be 100% ANA positive. However, it is more common to be on a drug such as procainamide (Pronestyl) or apresoline (Hydralazine) and have a drug-induced ANA without accompanying lupus-like symptoms. In patients with *Sjögren's syndrome*, about 80% are ANA positive. The frequency of ANA positivity in various rheumatic diseases is summarized below.

*ANA Positivity in Rheumatic Diseases**

Disease	*% ANA Positive*
Systemic lupus erythematosus	95-100%
Subacute cutaneous lupus	60-80%
Discoid lupus	4-10%
Drug-induced lupus	100%
MCTD	100%
Sjögren's syndrome	80%
Systemic sclerosis	60-95%
Polymyositis-dermatomyositis	50-75%
Rheumatoid arthritis	40-60%

*Ranges represent percentages found when using mouse kidney cells (less sensitive) or human epithelioid cell lines.

ANA SPECIFICITIES

The immunofluorescent test answers the question of whether the patient's serum has antinuclear antibodies but does not identify the nuclear component to which the autoantibody is directed. There are basically three reasons to obtain ANA specificities: (1) to help strengthen a particular clinical diagnosis since certain rheumatic diseases have distinct ANA specificities (see below); (2) to identify subsets of disease, for example, antibodies to SS-A/Ro are characteristically seen in certain subsets of patients with systemic lupus erythematosus and in certain patients with Sjögren's syndrome; and (3) to monitor disease activity. This is of limited usefulness since most ANAs do not change significantly with fluctuations of disease activity except for antibodies to double-stranded DNA, which in certain patients with lupus, particularly those with active lupus nephritis, correlate with disease activity. However, not all values do, depending on the method used for determining the titer.

Rheumatic Disease Associations with Antinuclear Antibodies

Specific ANA	*Rheumatic Disease Association*
Histone	Drug-induced LE
Sm	SLE
PCNA	SLE
centromere	limited scleroderma (CREST)
PM-1	polymyositis-scleroderma
Jo-1	polymyositis
SS-B/La	Sjögren's syndrome
SS-A/Ro	SLE and Sjögren's subsets
Scl-70	diffuse scleroderma

1. *Antibodies to DNA.* Antibodies to double-stranded DNA can be detected by a wide variety of techniques, including hemagglutination (which is a very sensitive but not a very specific method), radioimmunoassay, ELISA (enzyme-linked immunoabsorbent assay), and the *Crithidia lucilliae* immunofluorescence technique. Antibodies to double-stranded DNA are present in 60-70% of patients with systemic lupus erythematosus, usually in high levels. For example, using a radioimmunoassay, a greater than 30-40% binding (normal below 10%) often correlates with the presence of active systemic lupus erythematosus. However, although these antibodies may correlate with lupus activity, especially lupus nephritis, correlation has to be

established patient by patient on an *individual* basis. For example, there are patients who persistently have high levels of antibodies to double-stranded DNA but remain clinically quiescent.

It is also clear that not only the quantity of antibody to double-stranded DNA is important but also the quality of the antibody. IgG class anti-double-stranded DNA antibodies that are complement fixing are much more important in the pathogenesis of lupus nephritis than noncomplement fixing, IgM class anti-DNA antibodies. It is also important to realize that low titers of antibodies to double-stranded DNA may also be seen in other connective tissue diseases, so if a patient clinically "looks like scleroderma" but has low levels of antibodies to double-stranded DNA, the diagnosis is still scleroderma. Antibodies to single-stranded DNA are seen in both rheumatic and non-rheumatic diseases, and testing for these antibodies is of little clinical usefulness.

2. *Antibodies to Sm.* Antibodies to Sm are named after a patient, Smith, in whom this antibody system was first described. Antibodies to Sm are present in only 30% of all systemic lupus erythematosus patients but since these antibodies are rarely found in any other connective tissue disease, they are a highly specific disease marker for lupus. The presence of antibodies to Sm do not identify a subset of lupus patients. Therefore, they are of no prognostic significance.
3. *Antibodies to nRNP.* Antibodies to nuclear ribonuclear protein are seen in a wide variety of different connective tissue diseases. They occur in patients with lupus, scleroderma, rheumatoid arthritis, and Sjögren's syndrome, so they are not specific. However, the presence of these antibodies in high titer, coupled with the absence of antibodies to Sm or double-stranded DNA, is the serologic hallmark of the clinical overlap syndrome known as mixed connective tissue disease (MCTD), in which patients have clinically overlapping features of lupus, scleroderma, polymyositis, and, occasionally, rheumatoid arthritis. For example, 30% of patients with systemic lupus erythematosus will have antibodies to nRNP, but 100% of patients with mixed connective tissue disease will have antibodies to nRNP and in higher titer (by hemagglutination technique in the range of 1:10,000 to 1:100,000 or greater).
4. *Antibodies to SS-A/Ro and SS-B/La.* Antibodies to *SS-A/Ro* occur in a wide diversity of rheumatic diseases, although they occur most frequently in patients with either systemic lupus erythematosus or

Sjögren's syndrome. SS-A/Ro antibodies occur with increased frequency in certain *lupus disease subsets*: (1) SLE with thrombocytopenia, (2) "ANA-negative" lupus, (3) subacute cutaneous lupus, and (4) neonatal lupus (see below and Chapter 27 also).

SS-B/La antibodies occur in patients with primary Sjögren's syndrome and in Sjögren's syndrome associated with systemic lupus erythematosus. SS-A/Ro and/or SS-B/La antibodies are seen with increased frequency in extraglandular Sjögren's syndrome with vasculitis, central nervous system involvement or myositis. SS-A/Ro antibodies without SS-B/La antibodies are less specific for any particular connective tissue disease. They are seen not only in lupus and Sjögren's but also in patients with dermatomyositis, mixed connective tissue disease, and, sometimes, rheumatoid arthritis.

5. *Antibodies* to the *rheumatoid arthritis associated nuclear antigen (RANA)* are present in rheumatoid arthritis patients with or without associated Sjögren's syndrome. Unfortunately, antibodies to RANA have not been found to be clinically useful.

SEROLOGIC ASSOCIATIONS WITH SPECIFIC DISEASES

1. *Drug-Induced Lupus* (anti-histone antibodies)

   There are two drugs which are the major inducers of a lupus-like syndrome: procainamide (Pronestyl) and hydralazine (Apresoline), especially in slow acetylators, in whom the drug is less rapidly eliminated. Procainamide induces ANA positivity after approximately six to 12 months of use in about 50-75% of cases. Fortunately, only about 20% of these patients ever develop lupus-like symptoms. Hydralazine will induce ANA positivity in a smaller percentage (about 24-50%), and lupus-like symptoms occur in 8-13%. An interesting observation about drug-induced lupus is that it exhibits restricted clinical and serologic expression. Patients with drug-induced lupus usually present with arthralgias and pleuropericardial symptoms. Such features as renal involvement or central nervous system disease are not seen in drug-induced lupus.

   Serologically, patients with drug-induced lupus have antibodies to histones, but not to either double-stranded DNA or Sm which helps to distinguish them from patients with idiopathic lupus. Antihistone antibodies are also present in 25% of rheumatoid arthritis patients and less frequently in other connective tissue diseases. The pattern of immunofluorescence associated with anti-histone antibodies is homogeneous.

To implicate a drug in a lupus-like syndrome, the following guidelines are used: (1) a likely drug, (2) lupus-like features, (3) a positive ANA, usually homogeneous pattern in high titer, and (4) resolution of symptoms, and, subsequently, the positive ANA, after discontinuation of the drug. It should be noted that testing for anti-histone antibodies is interesting and of research importance, but is not critical in the diagnosis of drug-induced lupus.

2. *Progressive Systemic Sclerosis (Scleroderma)* (anti-Scl-70, anti-centromere, anti-nucleolar antigens)
   There are two specific ANAs that are serologic markers for scleroderma: antibodies to the Scl-70 antigen (topoisomerase I) and antibodies to centromere (kinetochore). *Antibodies to Scl-70* are found in only 20-25% of patients with progressive systemic sclerosis, but they are a specific disease marker for scleroderma since these antibodies are rarely found in any other disease. In particular, Scl-70 antibodies are a marker for the diffuse form of scleroderma.

   Antibodies to the centromere are found in a third of patients with progressive systemic sclerosis. When scleroderma patients are separated into those with the CREST variety (or limited scleroderma) and those with diffuse scleroderma, approximately 90-95% of patients with CREST syndrome will have antibodies to centromere as opposed to only 3% of patients with diffuse scleroderma. Therefore, antibodies to centromere appear to identify people with the CREST variety of scleroderma, which has a more benign course than that of diffuse scleroderma. Three nucleolar antigen-antibody systems have also been recently described in some scleroderma patients: antibodies to RNA polymerase I (4%), PM-Scl (3%) and fibrillarin (8%).
3. *Polymyositis-Dermatomyositis* (anti-PM-1, anti-Jo-1, anti-Mi-2)
   A number of precipitating antigen-antibody systems have been described in idiopathic polymyositis and dermatomyositis. There are three major systems. One is the PM system, also known as PM-Scl. Antibody to PM-1 recognizes a nucleolar antigen. This marker system appears to identify patients who are more likely to have overlapping features of polymyositis and scleroderma. Antibodies to Jo-1, which recognize histidyl t-RNA synthetase, are present in 30% of patients with polymyositis and particularly in polymyositis patients

with interstitial lung disease. Antibodies to PL-7 (threonyl tRNA synthetase) and PL-12 (alanyl tRNA synthetase) have also been described. Antibodies to Mi-2 are present in 25% of patients with dermatomyositis.

4. *Lupus Erythematosus*
Patients with SLE have a multiplicity of antinuclear antibodies, including antibodies to dsDNA (50-70%), ssDNA (70%), Sm (30%), nRNP (30%), SS-A/Ro (30%), SS-B/La (10-15%), histones (35-70%), PCNA (proliferating cell nuclear antigen) (7%), and Ku (10%). Some subsets show some ANA specificity.
   a) *Subacute cutaneous lupus* (SCLE) is a skin disease characterized by widespread, erythematous, scaly lesions on the face, neck, upper trunk, shoulders and extensor surfaces of the forearms (the sun-exposed areas). There are two forms: papulosquamous and annular. Approximately 50% of patients with subacute cutaneous lupus skin involvement will satisfy the ARA criteria for systemic lupus erythematosus. The serologic feature of SCLE is the presence of antibodies to SS-A/Ro and/or SS-B/La.
   b) *Neonatal lupus* is a rare condition in which neonates have discoid or subacute cutaneous lupus-like skin involvement with or without congenital heart block. The skin lesions are transient and resolve by six months of age, whereas the heart block is permanent and may require pacemaker placement. The mothers of children with neonatal lupus are often asymptomatic. If they do have symptoms, they are usually symptoms of either lupus or of Sjögren's syndrome. The common serologic feature of neonatal lupus is the presence of maternally-derived IgG antibodies to SS-A/Ro. Although antibodies to SS-A/Ro are the serologic marker of neonatal lupus, the vast majority of mothers who have antibodies to SS-A/Ro do not have children with neonatal lupus.

ANTI-PHOSPHOLIPID ANTIBODIES

Anti-phospholipid antibodies can be detected by the following methods: (1) a falsely positive serologic test for syphilis, (2) a lupus anticoagulant as determined by a prolonged partial thromboplastin time not corrected by normal plasma and confirmed to be due to a phospholipid inhibitor by such tests as platelet neutralization or the Russell viper venom test, or (3) an ELISA or radioimmunoassay determination of cardiolipin antibodies. Whether these methods measure the same or related phenomena is not clear, but the clinical correlates are the same.

Patients with anti-phospholipid antibodies are at increased risk for the following problems:

(1) arterial and venous thrombosis,
(2) recurrent spontaneous abortions,
(3) thrombocytopenia,
(4) focal neurologic manifestations of central nervous system lupus,
(5) fetal distress and/or demise in children of SLE mothers

Testing for the presence of anti-cardiolipin antibodies should be performed as part of the evaluation of young people with strokes or women with recurrent spontaneous abortions. The type and duration of treatment of the clinical manifestations of the "phospholipid syndrome" are currently being investigated in controlled trials. However, treatment of major thrombotic events should consist of long-term anticoagulation and there is suggestive evidence that treatment with prednisone and low-dose aspirin may result in a successful fetal outcome in habitual aborters who have anticardiolipin antibodies.

SUMMARY

The clinical immunology laboratory is a great help in diagnosing and following patients with rheumatic diseases. Understanding how the tests are performed and learning the strengths and weaknesses of the laboratory accessible to you are very important for the proper use of these tests.

SUGGESTED READINGS

1. Tan EM, Chan EKL, Sullivan KF, Rubin RL. Antinuclear antibodies (ANA's): diagnostically specific immune markers and clues toward the understanding of systemic autoimmunity. Clin Immunol Immunopathol. 1988; 47:121-41.

2. Harris EN, Phil M, Askerson RA, Hughes GRV. Antiphospholipid antibodies—autoantibodies with a difference. Ann Rev Med. 1988; 39:261-71.

3. Harmon CE. Antinuclear antibodies in autoimmune disease, significance and pathogenicity. Med Clin NA. 1985; 69:547-63.

Chapter 6

Joint Aspiration, Synovial Fluid Analysis and Intra-articular Injections

Needle aspiration of fluid from a symptomatic joint (arthrocentesis) is an important diagnostic and therapeutic tool. Many peripheral joints are easily accessible for arthrocentesis, while other deep and complex joints (e.g., the hip and spinal apophyseal joints) are best left to experts. Certain causes of acute and chronic joint arthritis are best diagnosed by arthrocentesis and include: septic joint, the crystal-induced arthropathies, and hemarthrosis. Therapeutic reasons for arthrocentesis include:

a. remove blood, pus, or large volumes of fluid from the joint that may be destructive or destabilizing, and
b. establish a route for intra-articular steroid injection.

A. GENERAL TECHNIQUE

1. *Arthrocentesis tray*
   The following items should be assembled prior to initiating the procedure. An adequate tray includes: alcohol sponges, iodine-containing swabs or solution, sterile gauzes, disposable syringes (3 ml to 30 ml), several 18- and 20-gauge needles, 27- or 25-gauge infiltrating needles, 1% lidocaine, appropriate steroid preparations, plain and heparinized test tubes, clean microscope slides with coverslips, ethyl chloride, plastic adhesive bandages and disposable latex gloves. If bacterial infection is suspected, it is optimal to have chocolate agar plates and aerobic and anerobic bacteria culture media available at bedside.

2. *Anatomic Visualization*
   Knowing the regional anatomy of the joint will not only minimize complications of the needle puncture but will add confidence and greatly improve chances of success. Reviewing the significant structural relationships around the joint space in *Gray's Anatomy,* the *Ciba Collection: Musculoskeletal* volume or other reference anatomy texts is recommended.
3. *Site Preparation and Aspiration*
   The patient should be fully informed on the reasons you are aspirating the joint as well as possible complications (pain, bleeding, and infection) and the general technique to be used. The patient should be reassured and given information throughout the procedure.
   a. With the joint in a stable and rested position, the landmarks described in the following section are identified. An impression is made over the proposed point of entry with a retracted ballpoint pen tip.
   b. The site is cleaned with an iodine containing solution and allowed to air dry.
   c. Sterile drapes and gloves are *not* necessary, although sterility at the site of puncture and of all materials penetrating the skin is absolutely crucial.
   d. Local anesthesia is optional but generally recommended. A small subcutaneous wheal of lidocaine is made with a 27- or 25-gauge needle. The needle is slowly advanced along the intended approach to the joint, depositing 1 to 1.5 ml of 1% lidocaine along the way. Alternatively, ethyl chloride may be used for surface anesthesia.
   e. Care must be taken throughout the procedure not to gouge the cartilage with needles.
   f. The infiltrating needle is withdrawn and an aspirating 20-gauge needle follows the anesthetized path to the joint space. Some of us prefer attaching *no* syringe to the aspirating needle. If you hold the hub of the needle like a throwing dart, the needle will be more maneuverable, and you can better feel various structures as the needle passes through or touches them than if a syringe is attached. Occasionally, the slight negative pressure caused by a syringe attached to

aspirating needle will occlude the needle lumen with synovium or debris and result in a false "dry" tap. If bone is hit, pull back slightly on the needle and redirect it.

g. Once the joint space is entered, fluid will appear at the hub of the needle, and a syringe can then be attached for aspiration. The aspiration should remove as much fluid as possible, but overly vigorous aspiration will cause bleeding and cartilage damage.

h. If large effusions are present (e.g., in a knee with large suprapatellar extension), an elastic support wrap (Ace bandage) should be applied prior to aspiration to insure optimal drainage. The wrap should begin at mid-thigh and proceed distally to the knee. Similar results can be obtained by having an assistant apply manual pressure over the suprapatellar pouch, popliteal area, or lateral recess of the knee to "milk" the effusion toward the aspirating needle.

B. APPROACHES TO SPECIFIC JOINTS AND BURSAE

1. *Knee*—With the knee comfortably extended in the supine position, the cephalad and caudal borders and the medial edge of the patella are determined. The puncture site for the medial approach is at the mid portion of the patella, 1 cm posterior to the

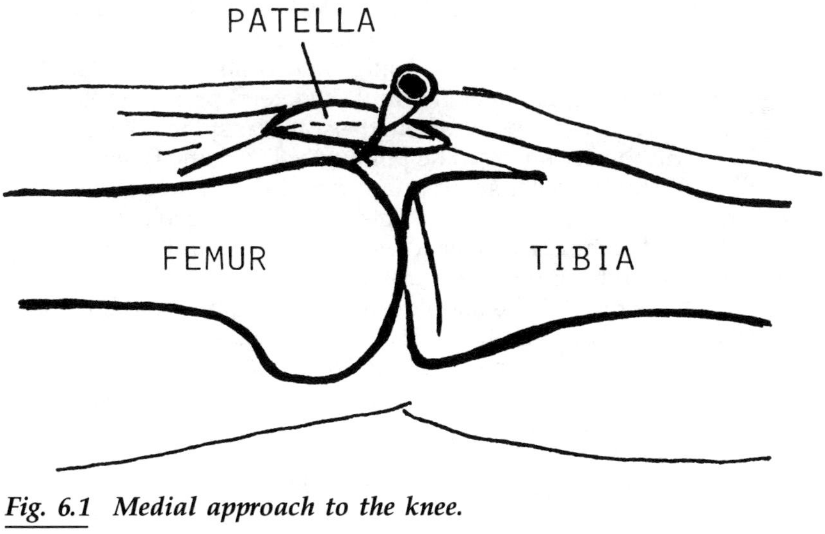

Fig. 6.1 Medial approach to the knee.

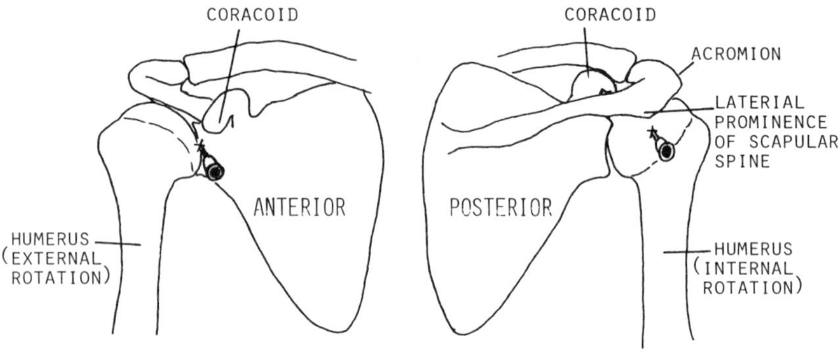

Fig. 6.2 Anterior and posterior approach to the shoulder.

patellar edge. The hub of the needle should be elevated 10-15 degrees from horizontal. The joint capsule is 1 to 2 cm beneath the skin surface. If the retropatellar space is narrow (chondromalacia or small fluid volume), the space can be slightly opened for easier access if downward pressure is applied to the lateral patellar margin.

2. *Shoulder*—The posterior approach is easy and nearly devoid of significant neurovascular obstacles. With the patient sitting comfortably, internally rotate the shoulder (ask the patient to place the fingers from the involved side in the contralateral axilla). Feel the scapular spine laterally until the lateral prominence is palpated. (This is the point where the scapular spine turns anterior to form the acromion). The point of entry is one fingerbreadth below this scapular spine prominence. Reach around and palpate the coracoid process anteriorly. The needle should be directed at the coracoid as it is slowly advanced. Proceed gently to avoid hitting bone or cartilage.

   Aspiration of the shoulder is also possible by the anterior approach. With the shoulder externally rotated, the point of entry is 1 to 1.5 cm below and 1 cm lateral to the coracoid process. The needle is directed posteriorly with a slight superior and lateral angulation.

3. *Ankle*—The patient is supine and the foot-leg angle is as close to 90° as comfortable. The point of entry is on the crease made over the tibial-talar joint when the foot is flexed. On this crease

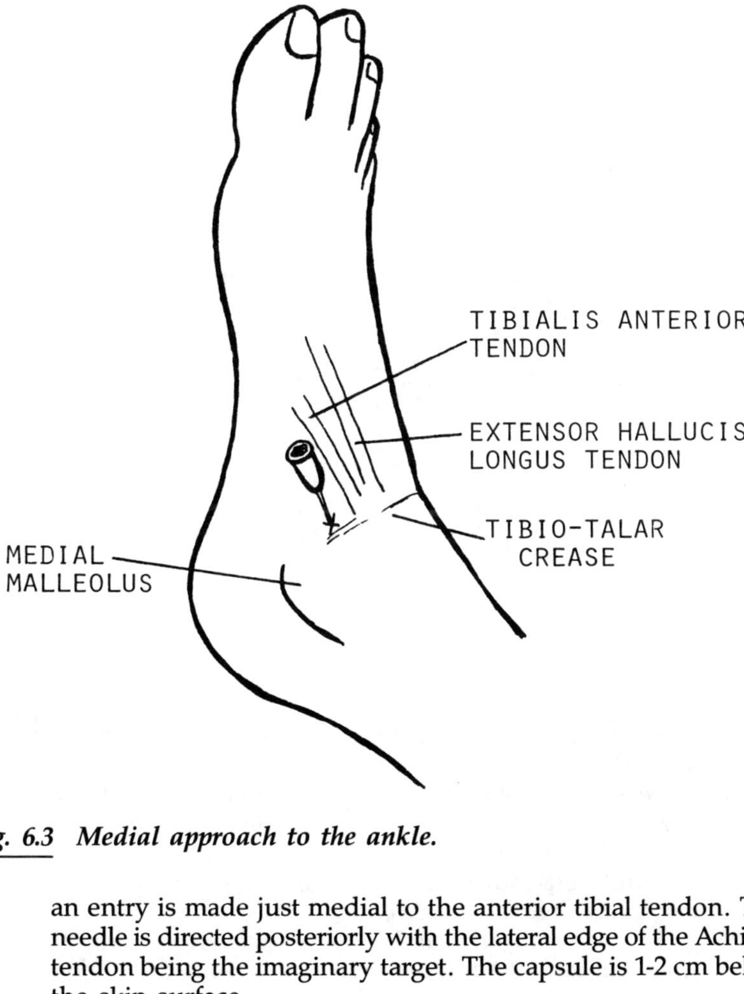

Fig. 6.3 Medial approach to the ankle.

an entry is made just medial to the anterior tibial tendon. The needle is directed posteriorly with the lateral edge of the Achilles tendon being the imaginary target. The capsule is 1-2 cm below the skin surface.

4. *Wrist*—The best approach to the wrist joint is dorsal since it avoids most neurovascular structures. The point of entry is just distal to the radius and just lateral to the extensor pollicis longus tendon. The wrist should be slightly flexed (resting over a small rolled towel) and the needle directed perpendicularly. If bone

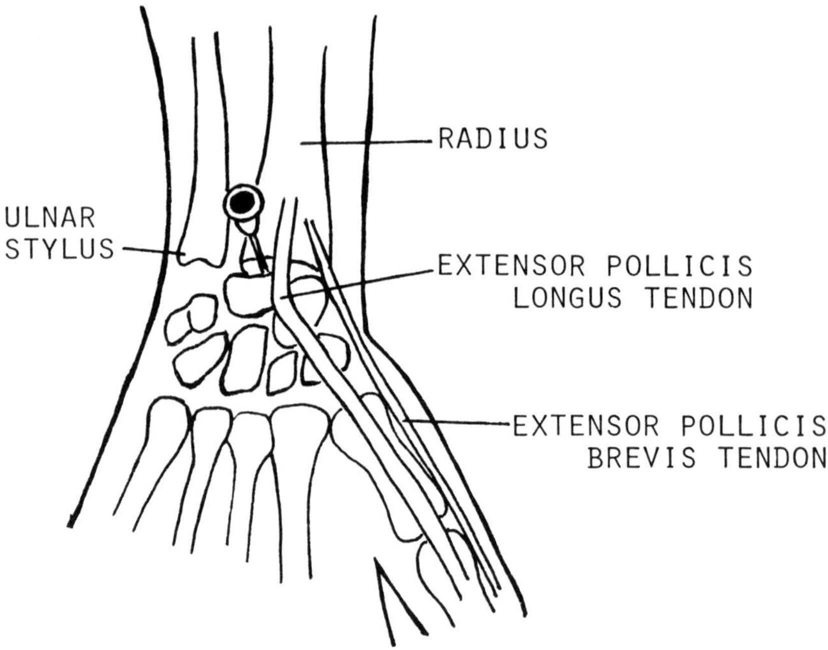

Fig. 6.4 Dorsal approach to the wrist.

is encountered at 0.5 to 1 cm, withdraw and redirect slightly toward the thumb.

5. *Elbow*—The safest approach into the elbow joint is laterally with the elbow flexed at 90 degrees. The point of entry is just inferior to the lateral humeral epicondyle with the needle directed medially and perpendicular to the skin. The joint space is 1 to 1.5 cm below the skin surface.
6. *Metacarpophalangeal and interphalangeal joints.* With the joint slightly flexed, the approach is either dorsomedial or dorsolateral into the joint capsule. Directing the needle between the articular surfaces is not necessary and may be damaging. Instead, the needle is gently guided beneath the extensor tendon. A small needle (23- to 25-gauge) will minimize trauma.
7. *Metatarsophalangeal joint.* The first MTP joint is not easily accessible, but it is frequently a joint requiring aspiration. The best

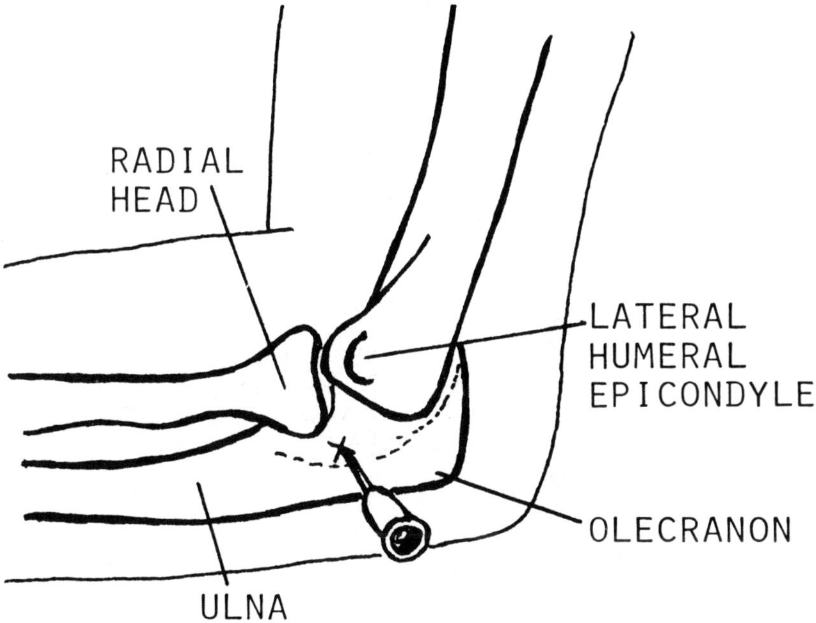

Fig. 6.5 *Lateral approach to the elbow.*

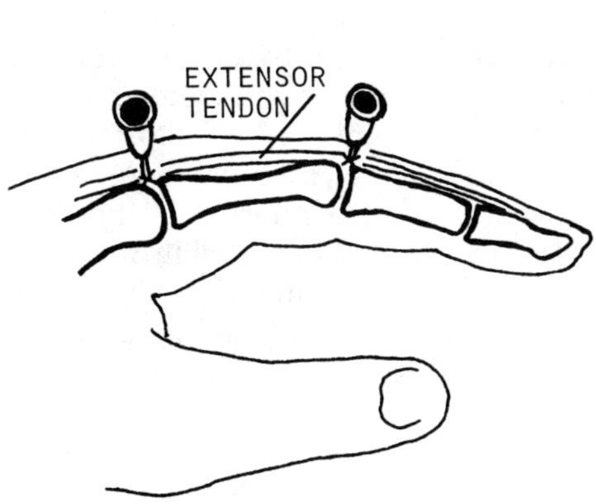

Fig. 6.6 *Aspiration of a small joint of the hand.*

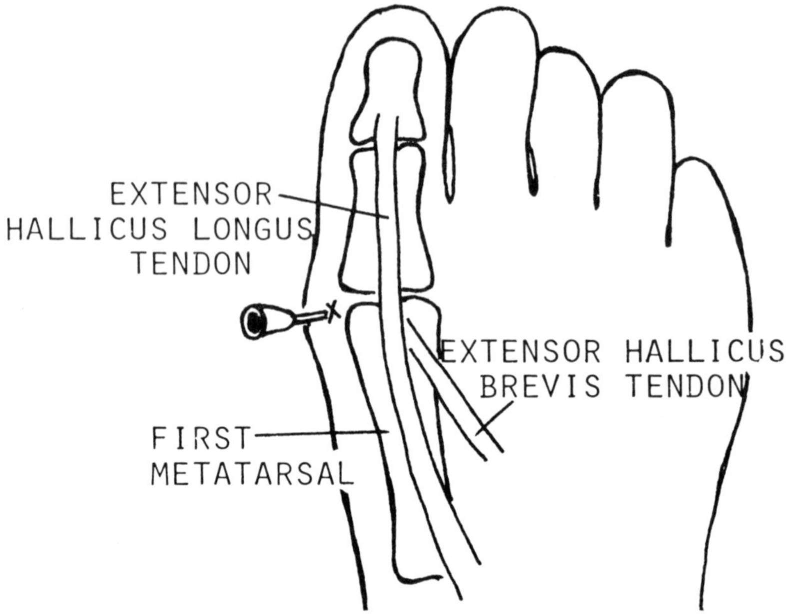

Fig. 6.7 Dorsomedial approach to the first MTP.

approach is dorsomedial with a 22-gauge needle directed under the extensor tendon. In patients with acute gout, local skin anesthesia with lidocaine is poorly tolerated and of little benefit. Instead a "quick numbing" with sprayed ethyl chloride may be used. A small volume (1 ml) of sterile saline should be available for injection and reaspiration in the case of a dry tap.

8. *Subdeltoid bursa.* This easily accessible bursa may be responsible for "impingement pain" when the shoulder is abducted. The point of entry is in the lateral midline of the shoulder, one fingerbreadth below the edge of the acromion. The needle is inserted under the acromial edge in a slightly cephalad direction.
9. *Other joints and bursae.* Other joints may occasionally be aspirated or injected, but, due to their deep location (e.g., hip) or their proximity to important structures (e.g., temporomandibular joint), are best left to experienced hands. Other

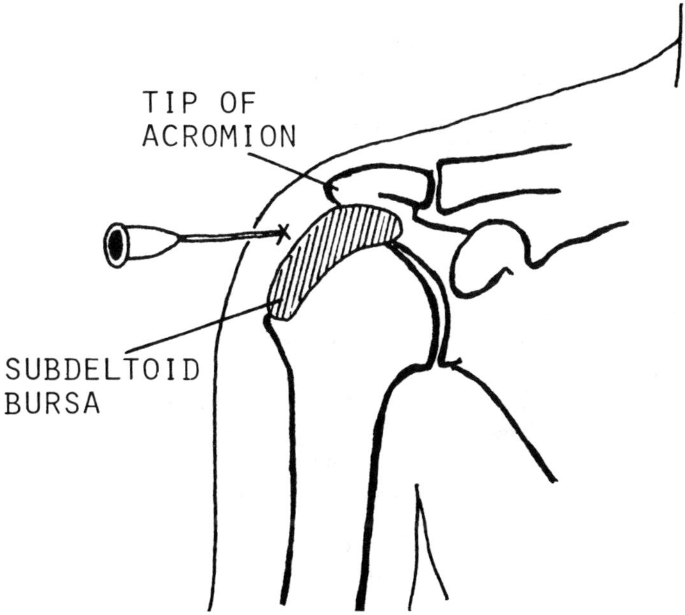

Fig. 6.8 Lateral approach to the subdeltoid bursa.

bursae and tendon sheaths such as the trochanteric bursa of the hip, the anserine bursa of the knee, the carpal tunnel, tarsal tunnel, and biceps tendon are readily accessible, and techniques to inject them are contained in orthopedic or rheumatology texts. The olecranon bursa may become quite enlarged in rheumatoid arthritis, gout, or trauma. Aspirating this bursa is discouraged unless sepsis needs to be ruled out. Due to its closeness to the skin surface and its susceptibility to trauma, the olecranon bursa is at greater risk than most other joints or bursae to develop secondary infections following arthrocentesis.

C. SYNOVIAL FLUID ANALYSIS

Speed in analyzing joint or bursal fluid is important to minimize artifacts. Routine synovial fluid processing includes:

I. Gram stain and culture.

—fluid is promptly carried to the lab for aerobic and anaerobic cultures and gram stain. If mycobacterial or fungal infections are suspected, specific cultures should be obtained.

II. Wet mount for crystals
—fluid is placed on a clean microscope slide with a coverslip for brightfield and compensated polarized microscopy.

Compensated Polarized Appearance of Crystals

Crystals	Description	Birefringence
Monosodium urate	Needle-shaped	– (strong)
CPPD	Rhomboidal	+ (weak)
Basic calcium (hydroxyapatite)	"shiny coin" on brightfield	0
Lipids	Maltese cross	+
Injected steroids	Needle or pleomorphic	+ or –
Cholesterol plates	Very large geometric plates	+ or –

III. Leukocyte count and differential
—a heparinized tube with 1 or more cc of fluid is sent to the laboratory
—bursal fluid cell counts are much lower than those found in synovial fluid for a given condition (e.g., crystals, infection, etc.)

Classification of Synovial Fluid

Test	Normal	Non-inflammatory	Inflammatory	Septic*
Viscosity	good	good	poor	variable
Appearance	clear	clear yellow	cloudy yellow	purulent
WBC	200	200-2,000	2,000-75,000	40,000-100,000
PMN (%)	<25	<25	>50	>75

*Early or partially treated bacterial arthritis (or from a leukopenic patient) may appear as either inflammatory or non-inflammatory fluid.

IV. Other tests
—determination of appearance and viscosity should be made at the bedside.

—glucose, protein, complement, and LDH levels are rarely helpful.

D. INTRA-ARTICULAR CORTICOSTEROIDS

1. *Indications*

   Steroid injections may be useful as local palliative therapy for either degenerative or inflammatory arthritis in the following settings:

   a. when only one of several peripheral joints are inflamed
   b. to treat joints "resistant" to systemic anti-inflammatory therapy
   c. when systemic anti-inflammatory therapy is contraindicated
   d. as an adjunct to rehabilitation therapy.

2. *Contraindications*

   a. Absolute
      —septic arthritis or periarticular sepsis
      —bacteremia or cellulitis
      —unstable joint
   b. Relative
      —clotting disorder
      —juxta-articular osteoporosis
      —total joint arthroplasty
      —failure of prior injections

3. *Adverse Effects*

   Serious adverse reactions to intra-articular steroid injections are rare if proper technique and dosing schedules are observed.

   a. Infection: this most dreaded consequence occurs only once per 2,000-15,000 injections in most series.
   b. Post-injection flare: occurs in 2-5% of injections. Characterized by heat, swelling, and pain and typically occurs 4 to 8 hours post injection. Symptoms persist for 3 to 48 hours and can be treated with oral analgesics. This is more likely to occur with the less soluble steroid preparations (e.g., Triamcinolone).

4. *Administration*

   Repeat injection of the same joint may be performed safely if limited to no more often than every four to six months. Whether or not anesthetics are also injected, the joint should ideally be immobilized and non-weight bearing for 24 to 72 hours.

Immobilization will enhance the duration of symptomatic improvement.

5. *Intra-articular Steroid Preparations*
   This is a partial listing of commonly used steroids.

Steroid Preparation	*Relative Equivalents*
Dexamethasone sodium phosphate (Decadron) 4 mg/ml	5.2
Betamethasone sodium phosphate (Celestone) 4 and 6 mg/ml	5.2
Methylprednisolone acetate (Depo-Medrol) 20, 40, and 80 mg/ml	1.0
Triamcinolone acetonide (Kenalog) 10 and 40 mg/ml	1.0
Tramcinolone diacetate (Aristocort) 40 mg/ml	1.0
Triamcinolone hexacetonide (Aristospan) 20 mg/ml	1.0
Prednisolone tebutate (Hydeltra-T.B.A.)	0.8

6. *Dosage*
   The dose of steroids and the volume injected varies with the size of the joint.

Size of Joint	*Dose of Steroid**	*Volume***
Large	24-40 mg	2-2 ml
Medium	15-25 mg	0.5-1 ml
Small	2.5-10 mg	0.1-0.5 ml

*Expressed in methylprednisolone equivalents

**This volume includes steroid plus anesthetic. Long acting (insoluble) steroids should not be mixed with anesthetics containing paraben preservatives.

SUGGESTED READINGS

1. Owen DS, Irby R. Intra-articular and soft-tissue aspiration and injection. Clin Rheumatol Practice. 1986; 4:52.

2. Gray RG, Tenenbaum J, Gottlieb NL. Local corticosteroid injection treatment in rheumatoid arthritis. Sem Arthritis Rheum. 1981; 10:231-54.

3. Goldenberg DL. Synovial fluid analysis in current practice. Postgrad Adv Rheumatol. 1987; 2:1.

Chapter 7

The Radiology of Articular Disorders

A. WHY ORDER "X-RAYS?"

The use of radiographs and other imaging techniques is crucial in the evaluation and management of rheumatic disorders. The type of radiographic abnormalities being sought include: soft tissue swelling and calcification, osteoporosis, reactive bone formation, cartilage space narrowing, bone erosions, and joint malalignment or ankylosis. It is also important to note the distribution of joint abnormalities. The combination of characteristic radiographic changes with a particular pattern of involvement can frequently lead to exact radiologic diagnosis.

Radiographs are helpful in determining the extent and severity of disease. This is important in deciding whether the source of joint pain is *inflammatory* with relative preservation of articular surfaces or *mechanical* ("bone on bone") pain with severe destruction of joint architecture. Serial radiographs may also be used to monitor disease progression and effectiveness of therapies.

B. WHEN TO ORDER "X-RAYS?"

While radiographs are very helpful in Rheumatology, they are also expensive and expose patients to radiation. The diagnostic value of radiography depends on when in the clinical course of a particular disease they are obtained. Radiographic changes of septic joints may occur in several days (staphylococcus), in days to weeks (gonococcus), or over years (tuberculosis). It is unusual for the x-ray changes of rheumatoid arthritis to occur in the first four or five months of symptoms. Gouty changes may not occur until after five to six acute episodes (over three to four years). On the other hand,

sacroiliac x-ray changes are usually already evident by the time ankylosing spondylitis symptoms occur. When and how often we obtain joint radiographs will depend on the disease(s) being considered in the differential.

C. WHAT TO ORDER?

1. *Plain films.* Plain radiographs should be the initial radiographic approach to bone and joint symptoms. The joint is usually viewed in two projections so that early changes won't be missed. The commonly requested projections are:

Hand/Wrist	Foot
PA	PA
Oblique	Lateral
Shoulder	Knee
AP (ext. rot.)	Standing AP
AP (int. rot.)	Lateral
Hip	Sacroiliac
AP	Mod. Ferguson

In mono- (or oligo-) articular disease, comparison films of the uninvolved, contralateral joint will help determine the level of osteopenia, subtle changes in joint space narrowing, and the presence of normal variants of bone formation.

In polyarticular disease, the radiographic survey is tailored to the joints with most severe symptoms and longest duration. Also, consideration is given to where the most diagnostic changes are likely to occur for the particular disease. Knowing the *distribution* and *type* of destructive lesions is therefore important.

2. *Bone scintigraphy.* Bone scans are frequently used to confirm the presence of disease in patients with mild or intermittent joint symptoms. Bone scans can also be used to demonstrate the pattern of involvement and to assess disease activity. Osteomyelitis may be detected by comparing scans taken immediately and two hours after isotope injection. If there is a high index of suspicion for fracture, the bone scan is often diagnostic in the face of negative plain films. A radiographically detectable callus takes 10-14 days to develop.
3. *Conventional tomography.* Plain tomograms are still a good way to evaluate certain complex joints. These include the temporo-

mandibular, the sternoclavicular, and the costovertebral joints.

4. *Computed tomography* (CT). The role of CT in musculoskeletal evaluation is not yet clear. Several areas where it does appear to have advantages over conventional radiographs are osteonecrosis of the hip (aseptic necrosis), early sacroiliitis, spinal stenosis, apophyseal joint arthritis, and disc herniation.
5. *Magnetic Resonance Imaging* (MRI). MRI has the great advantage of defining not only the skeletal structures but also soft tissue elements such as cartilage, tendons, ligaments, synovium, and spinal cord without the use of contrast media. While the full usefulness of this technique in the musculoskeletal work-up is still evolving, it is already widely used to evaluate the cervical spine in rheumatoid arthritis and for detecting early changes of avascular necrosis of the hip.
6. *Arthrography.* The injection of radiocontrast material into a joint can help identify certain soft tissue abnormalities, such as popliteal (Baker's) cyst of the knee, rotator cuff tear, or meniscal cartilage tear. During arthrocentesis of deep structures such as the hip joint, a small volume of contrast is injected through a fluoroscopically guided needle to ensure proper needle placement.

D. CHARACTERISTIC PATTERNS OF INVOLVEMENT

The distribution of joint destruction can be helpful in determining the disease process—especially early in the disease course. The typical patterns for common rheumatic diseases are described below.

1. *Rheumatoid Arthritis* (RA). Bilateral symmetry of involvement is characteristic. Frequently involved joints are: small joints of hands and feet (MCPs, PIPs, and MTPs), wrists (carpal bones and ulnar styli), cervical spine ($C_{1\text{-}2}$ and $C_{4\text{-}6}$), and knees (symmetric loss of medial, lateral, and retropatellar spaces). Also involved are hips, shoulders, and elbows.
2. *Osteoarthritis* (OA). Asymmetry of involvement is characteristic. Frequently involved joints are hands (DIPs, PIPs, and first carpal-metacarpal), cervical spine (especially $C_{3\text{-}7}$), lumbar spine, hips, knees (asymmetric loss of either medial or lateral space), and feet (especially first MTP).
3. *Ankylosing Spondylitis* (AS). Axial skeletal and large peripheral joints (particularly the lower extremities) are primarily affected. Sacroiliac joints are usually involved early with bilateral changes

of irregular joint space with sclerosis. The lumbar, thoracic, and cervical spine may be involved with squaring of anterior vertebral bodies and syndesmophyte formation resulting in the "bamboo" spine. Hips, knees, and shoulders may show changes similar to RA. The pubic symphysis may also be involved.

4. *Reiters' Syndrome (RS) and Psoriatic Arthritis (PA).* Asymmetry helps distinguish these diseases from RA. Predilection for a particular "ray" or a hand or foot is commonly seen so that the worse changes may occur in the DIP, PIP, and MCP of a single digit. Sacroiliac involvement is usually unilateral and distinguishes these diseases from AS. Spinal involvement with RS and PA is characterized by large asymmetric "non-marginal" syndesmophytes.
5. *Gout.* Early changes usually occur in the first, second, and fifth MTPs. Later stages of gout may involve any joint but especially the hands (PIPs and DIPs), wrists, midfoot, elbows, and knees.
6. *Calcium Pyrophosphate Deposition Disease (CPPD) or Pseudogout.* The distribution of radiographic changes is similar to OA. Chondrocalcinosis (calcified cartilage) is most frequently observed in the knees, shoulders, and wrists (especially in the ulnar-carpal space).

RADIOLOGIC APPEARANCE OF COMMON RHEUMATIC DISEASE

The drawings in Figure 7.1 (p. 54) represent the characteristic radiographic changes that appear in the small joints of certain common rheumatic conditions. Similar changes may also be present in large joints. The "bare" areas of a joint are where bones are covered by synovium but not cartilage. These are usually the earliest sites of erosions caused by proliferative synovitis (as in rheumatoid arthritis).

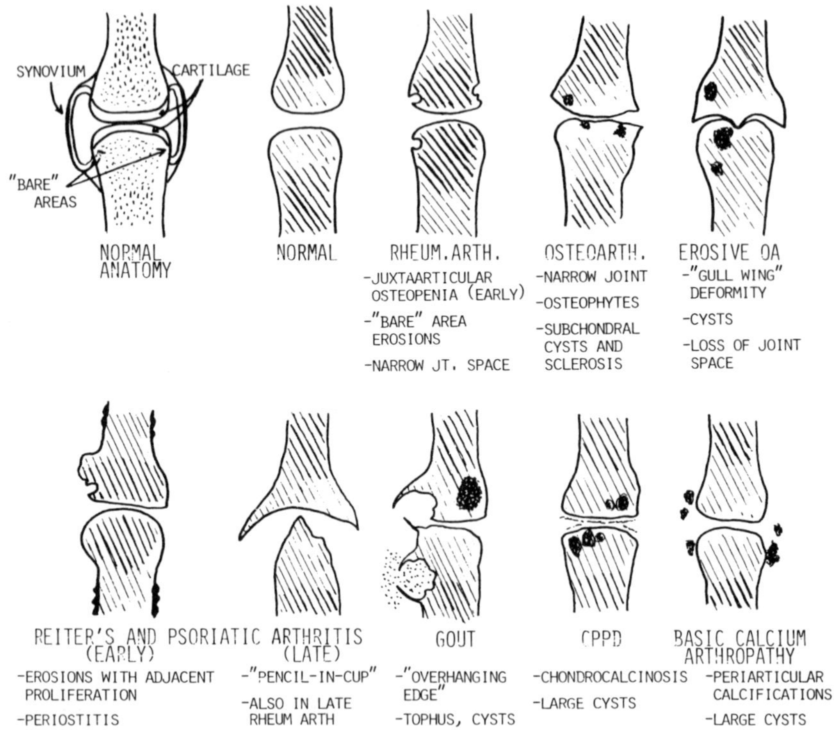

Fig. 7.1

SUGGESTED READINGS

1. Forrester DM, Brown JC (editors). Radiological investigation in rheumatology. Clin Rheum Dis. 1983; 9:289-483.

2. Resnick D, Niwayama G. *Diagnosis of Bone and Joint Disorders.* 2nd edition, Philadelphia: W. B. Saunders Co., 1987.

3. Gillespy T, Genant H, Helms CA. Magnetic resonance imaging of osteonecrosis. Radiol Clin North Am 1986; 24:193-204.

Chapter 8

Common Disease Patterns and Associations

Learning the patterns of joint involvement and recruitment, associated involvement of other organs, and the time course of various rheumatic diseases is necessary before one is able to recognize the correct diagnosis and provide appropriate therapy. The number of joints involved, predominance of large vs. small joints, upper vs. lower extremities, presence of serological abnormalities such as rheumatoid factor and antinuclear antibodies, association of peripheral arthritis and spondylitis, age and sex of the patient, and association with various extraarticular manifestations all contribute to our ability to diagnose the condition. When dealing with the more systemic rheumatic conditions, the specific organ involvement and sequence of disease manifestations become useful. This chapter will briefly describe various patterns and common associations that will allow you to recognize diagnostic features.

A. IMPORTANT DEFINITIONS

Joint Involvement: This can be classified in several ways,

By *number*: monoarticular = one joint
oligo- or pauciarticular = two to four joints
polyarticular = five or more joints.

By *symmetry*: symmetrical = same joints bilaterally
asymmetrical = involvement in one or more joints in one side and different joints on the opposite side

By *recruitment*: additive or cumulative = ongoing inflammation in one or more joints while additional joints are becoming involved.
migratory = inflammation resolves completely in between attacks.

By *specific joints*: large vs. small, upper vs. lower extremity

By *temporal characteristics*: acute, subacute or chronic. These terms have implications of intensity as well as duration.

B. SYNDROMES ASSOCIATED WITH SPECIFIC PATTERNS OF JOINT INVOLVEMENT

1. *Acute-monoarticular arthritis*

The differential diagnosis of acute monoarticular arthritis includes septic arthritis, crystalline arthropathies such as gout, pseudogout, and calcium hydroxyapatite disease, inherited problems such as coagulopathies (for example, hemophilia), trauma, and/or an atypical presentation of a disease with usual polyarticular or oligoarticular involvement (rheumatoid arthritis, Reiter's syndrome, etc.). A basic tenet to follow when only *one* joint is acutely inflamed is that it is *septic* until *proven* otherwise. Therefore, the most important diagnostic test to do in a patient with monoarticular arthritis is joint aspiration to look for infection. Gram stain and cultures should be done for both bacteria and fungi, and a synovial fluid white cell count and differential should be determined. The cell count is useful to follow the response to therapy. In addition, the synovial fluid should be examined under polarized light for crystals.

If the acute monoarticular arthritis is due to infection, early institution of antibiotic therapy combined with repeated joint aspirations is essential to prevent joint damage. If the monoarticular arthritis is traumatic due to torn menisci or ligaments or to osteonecrosis, the fluid will be bloody. Without a history of trauma, bloody fluid should suggest the possibility of a coagulopathy or villonodular synovitis, or rarely, metastatic tumor. Appropriate tests of coagulation, fluid cytology, or biopsy will establish the cause. It is important to remember that there may be more than one cause for the acute monoarticular arthritis; for example, a septic joint may be superimposed on an osteoarthritic or rheumatoid joint.

2. *Chronic Monoarticular Arthritis*

A more chronic monoarticular arthritis is more likely due to an indolent fungal or mycobacterial infection or to ongoing low-grade synovitis from crystals or overuse. The specific joint involved can be very helpful in suggesting the diagnosis. Acute inflammation of the first MTP, "podagra," is often due to gout, although psoriatic arthritis and calcific tendonitis may also present like this. In some patients, the inflammation becomes chronic.

3. *Symmetrical Polyarthritis*
   Rheumatoid arthritis patients classically develop and often present with small symmetrical joint involvement of the hands and feet (metacarpal phalangeal joints, metatarsal phalangeal joints, and proximal interphalangeal joints). In contrast, the arthritis of patients with psoriasis, Reiter's syndrome, and other spondyloarthropathies usually evolves into an asymmetric pattern involving large joints most often in the lower extremities (knees, ankles, and hind foot). The small joints of the hands and feet are rarely involved in these diseases.

   In contrast, the small peripheral joints are classically involved in rheumatoid arthritis and systemic lupus erythematosus. These diseases occur more frequently in women (approximate 3:1 ratio), while ankylosing spondylitis and Reiter's produce symptoms predominantly in males. Viral arthritis may also present with symmetrical small joint involvement but is usually short lived (days to weeks).
4. *Additive and Migratory Patterns*
   The pattern of recruitment of inflamed joints may also give clues as to the etiology of the arthritis. The most common pattern of joint involvement in patients with chronic inflammatory polyarthritis like rheumatoid arthritis is additive or cumulative. In contrast, patients with rheumatic fever or gonococcal arthritis often have a migratory pattern. This means that the inflammatory changes and pain in one joint may remit while simultaneously other joints are becoming inflamed. The joint inflammation in patients with migratory arthritis tends to peak in 12-24 hours and subside in 2-5 days.
5. *Intermittent arthritis*
   This is seen in gout, pseudogout, pallindromic rheumatism, familial Mediterranean fever (recurrent polyserositis), and sarcoidosis, among others. Once the acute attack subsides, the patient experiences no pain or residual problems in that joint until the next attack, which may occur years later. In untreated gout, the initial intermittent pattern may slowly evolve over many years into an additive pattern.

   Knowing the time course of the various arthritides also aids in making diagnoses. In acute gout, the arthritis pain and inflammation peak within a few hours. If untreated, pain will gradually subside over 7 to 10 days. Septic arthritis may peak more slowly than gout, and instead of subsiding gradually, pain becomes progressively more severe as cartilage is ultimately damaged if the infection is not treated. If the infected joint is treated, the arthritis and pain should subside. Rheumatoid arthritis and other chronic polyarthritides cause a "sine" wave pattern of exacerbations and improvement superimposed upon a baseline of ongoing arthritis activity.

The specific joints involved also provide clues to the diagnosis. For example, involvement mostly limited to the second and third MCPs, wrists, and knees is very suggestive of hemochromatosis, especially in males in the fifth decade. A pattern of shoulder, wrists, knees, and fingers, especially with prominent shoulder involvement, is characteristic of amyloid arthropathy.

6. *Pain with weight-bearing or at rest*
In general, acutely inflamed joints are very painful even at rest. Such joints tend to produce a sharp, throbbing, exquisite type of pain. Patients with gout or septic arthritis cannot tolerate pressure or bear weight on the painful inflamed joint. In contrast, chronically inflamed joints and mechanical problems secondary to degenerative changes produce a constant, dull, achy pain present with rest or use. If superimposed degenerative arthritis complicates a chronically inflamed joint, use and weight-bearing may exacerbate the pain.

SUMMARY

If one is able to understand these basic tenets of classification, organizing one's approach to the differential diagnosis of various arthritides would be easy. It should not be necessary to consider all the types of arthritis when a patient presents with a typical pattern of joint involvement.

SUGGESTED READINGS

1. Schumacher HR Jr., Klippel JH, Robinson DR. *Primer on the rheumatic diseases*, ninth edition. Atlanta: Arthritis Foundation, 1988.

2. Kelley WN, Harris ED Jr, Ruddy S, Sledge CB. *Textbook of Rheumatology,* third edition. Philadelphia: W.B. Saunders Co. 1989.

3. McCarty D, editor. *Arthritis and Allied Conditions—A Textbook,* 11th edition. Philadelphia: W.B. Saunders Co., 1989.

Chapter 9

Making the Diagnosis of a Rheumatic Disease—Relevant Concepts of Clinical Epidemiology

Whenever we evaluate a patient, we can reach any one of four possible conclusions, depending on whether or not the patient truly has the disease. This is illustrated below in Table 9.1.

Table 9.1.
Conclusions possible after evaluating a patient

	Disease	
	Present	*Absent*
We conclude the disease is present	a True Positive	b False Positive
We conclude the disease is absent	c False Negative	d True Negative

Conclusion a—*True Positive*: The patient has the disease and we correctly determine this to be the case. If we can prescribe effective, non-morbid treatment, the patient should feel and do better.

Conclusion b—*False positive*: The patient does not have the disease, though he or she may think so and we agreed. Both the patient and we are in trouble!

Conclusion c—*False negative*: The patient has the disease but we wrongly determine otherwise. The patient will go undiagnosed and untreated.

Conclusion d—*True negative*: Both we and the facts concur. Now we still need to determine what other condition is responsible for the patient's complaints.

The judgment call associated with reaching the right conclusion of whether or not a given patient has a rheumatic disease or syndrome depends on our ability to perform the following steps.

1. *Recognize symptoms and signs* suggestive of a specific disease. We do this mostly through the process of pattern recognition.
2. *Know the usefulness and limitations* of symptoms, signs, diagnostic tests, and other findings associated with the presence of the disease.
3. *Determine the likelihood* that the specific disease is present, given the presence or absence of specific symptoms, signs, and test results in any given patient.

The ability with which we can do all the steps above determines how successful we are at doctoring. The science of medicine that teaches us how to evaluate diagnostic findings and therapeutic strategies is known as *clinical epidemiology.* The concepts of clinical epidemiology involved in the steps listed above are the topic of this chapter.

I. Recognition of Pattern of Illness or Disease

This is what our textbooks are all about. We have discussed some of these patterns in earlier chapters and will provide in later chapters more in-depth descriptions of the complaints, the physical and laboratory findings present in association with each particular illness, and the expected outcome of the illness with and without therapy. The more familiar we are with each disease entity or clinical syndrome, the more likely we are to make the diagnosis early and correctly. However, recognition of disease assumes that we can elicit a reliable history and perform an accurate physical examination. In fact, symptoms may or may not be elicited at varying times from the same patient, depending on the patient's reliability and recall, the physician's ability to ask the necessary questions, and/or the stage of the illness. Likewise, physical findings may be grossly obvious to all, subtle and difficult to find except to a few, or simply imagined because of our expectation that they should be present. Two or more observers often differ in their assessment of whether a finding is present or not, and this is most likely to occur if the finding is unexpected or of mild dimensions.

Such discrepancies in the history and clinical findings can be due to variation in several factors. The *variation may be biologic*—for example, edema of the ankles is more likely to be present after the patient is upright for some time; or the discrepant findings may be due to *observer* or *subject* variation. Safeguards we can use to limit observer or subject variation include repetitive training of observers, and standardizing the conditions under which the historical, physical, or laboratory findings are elicited. The better we get at correctly eliciting symptoms and signs, the more likely it is that our findings will be reproducible and accurate.

II. Evaluation of the Usefulness and Limitations of Diagnostic Tests

Recognizing the illness or diseases implies the ability to define it. To do this, we often have to rely on development of the illness over time into well-advanced classic disease. Other times, we use histopathologic diagnoses based on biopsy or autopsy findings. In clinical practice, we often do not wish to wait for the disease to advance before making a diagnosis and instituting treatment, so we are forced to use clinical, laboratory, and radiologic findings associated with the suspected illness to make the diagnosis. The usefulness and limitations of these diagnostic findings are discussed below.

An ideal finding—be it a part of the history, a physical finding, or a test result, should be both *valid* (or accurate) and *reliable* (or reproducible) and *subject to little or no variation*. In addition, the finding should always be present in patients with the disease and absent in those without it, such as the joint is, or is not, inflamed. If the finding is reported in an ordered scale like 1+ to 4+ inflammation, or in actual numbers (e.g., mg/dl), the separation of findings in patients with the disease compared to healthy individuals or patients with other diseases should be very clear. Unfortunately, real findings almost always overlap to some extent between these two groups. Which findings or values are considered normal and which abnormal depends on the degree of overlap between the sick and well populations and whether we are more interested in identifying all patients with disease (*ruling in*) or in making sure a patient does not have the disease (*ruling out*).

> *Exercise #1—Diagnosing SLE*
> Let us say that we want to know sensitivity and specificity (also called operating characteristics) of the fluorescent antinuclear antibody (ANA) test in identifying patients with systemic lupus erythematosus (SLE). To do this, we use the test in 100 patients who we know have SLE and in 100 medical students and lab technicians who are not supposed to have the disease. We run the subject's serum undiluted and at twofold dilutions from 1:10 to 1:2560. Let us say we find that the titer of serum at which we can best separate these two groups is 1:80. Using this titer of 1:80 or greater as indicative of the presence of SLE, we find that 66 of the patients with lupus among the 100 we tested have a positive or abnormal finding. This means that the test, when positive at a serum dilution of 1:80 or greater, has a *sensitivity* of 66% since it can identify 66% of the SLE patients (*true positives*). Its *false negative* rate is 34% (100% − sensitivity). (Substrate used for ANA is mouse kidney.)
>
> Among the controls, we find that only 20 of 100 test positive at 1:80 or above, therefore, the test is appropriately negative in 80%, that is, its *specificity* is 80%. Its *false positive* rate is 20% (100% − specificity). Knowing the sensitivity and specificity of the test and the number of SLE patients and controls tested, we can construct a 2 x 2 table like the one below.

How come we obtained these findings? You have heard the ANA is a very sensitive test, how can we say it is only 66% sensitive?

The reason is that we chose a cut-off titer of 1:80 as the "abnormal" or *positive result*. If we wanted to increase the test's sensitivity so that it would identify nearly all lupus patients, we would change the cut-off and choose a serum titer of 1:10 or undiluted as an abnormal test. In this case, the sensitivity would increase to 95%. However, by doing this we would also lose specificity since many more healthy controls may have a positive ANA in such a minuscule titer, and the specificity would decrease from 80 to 60%.

Table 9.2
Characteristics of a positive ANA of 1:80 or higher
Prevalence of SLE in the population tested = 50%,
Sensitivity = 66%, Specificity = 80%

		SLE *Present*	*Absent*	
ANA titer of 1:80 or higher	*Present*	66 (true +)	20 (false +)	86 total + tests + predictive value = 66/86×100 = 77%
	Absent	34 (false −)	80 (true −)	114 total − tests − predictive value = 80/114x100 = 70%
		100 SLE patients	100 healthy controls	200 total subjects

(Use of a human epithelioid cell line would also increase the sensitivity—see Chapter 5).

WARNING #1: For a given test, *any change* in *cutoff value* that *increases* the *sensitivity* is *off-set* by a *decrease in specificity.* Likewise, any *increase in specificity* is accompanied by a *decrease in sensitivity.* This DOES NOT mean that all tests that are more sensitive must be less specific. The *sensitivity and specificity* of each test are characteristics unique to that particular test. What it does mean is that, *for any given test,* changing the value used as "abnormal" changes the sensitivity and specificity of that test.

An ideal test would be 100% sensitive so it could identify all patients with the disease without missing any as false negatives. It would also be 100% specific so it could identify as negative all controls and produce no false positives. Unfortunately, no symptom, sign, or test finding has perfect operating characteristics, with the exception of some autopsy findings like presence of metastatic cancer or some arbitrary values like "anemia" if the serum hemoglobin is below 12 gm/dl.

WARNING #2: Diagnostic tests are usually evaluated in patients with the disease and compared to findings in *healthy* controls. In clinical practice, however, they are evaluated in ill patients with clinical characteristics similar to those of the disease being ruled out. Therefore, in the clinical situation, the specificity of the test is likely to change, since the test results are more likely to overlap between these two more similar populations.

III. Assessment of Disease Probability in the Presence of an Abnormal Finding

Once you know the findings in your particular patient, the chances or probability that the patient has the disease can be estimated if you know (or can accurately guess) the likely prevalence. *Prevalence* is the total number of individuals with the disease expected or found in given populations at given points in time. *Incidence* is the number of *new* cases of the disease that occur during a certain time period. Prevalence depends on the incidence of the disease and its clinical course. If a disease is short-lived because of short duration of illness or frequent untimely death, the prevalence will be lower than for a disease that may have a lower incidence but a longer duration of illness and lower mortality. Knowing the likely prevalence of the disease in the population you are testing gives you an estimate of the *pre-test* probability of disease in your patient.

Exercise #2: Meaning of an abnormal ANA in a symptomatic or ill population.
Let's go back to our earlier 2 × 2 table for ANA results and presence of SLE (see Table 9.2). Among all 200 individuals tested, the pre-test probability of SLE or prevalence was 50% since 100 of the 200 individuals tested were patients with SLE. Among the 86 with a positive test, 66 had SLE. Therefore, the likelihood of SLE, given a positive ANA of 1:80 or higher in this population of 200 individuals with a prevalence of SLE of 50%, is 66/86 x 100 or 77%. This *positive predictive value* (also known as the post-test probability) varies depending on the prevalence (or pre-test probability) of the disease in the popu-

lation you test. In this population with a prevalence of 50%, an abnormal test (positive ANA of 1:80 or higher) would have a 77% likelihood of being due to presence of SLE.

Exercise #3: Screening asymptomatic populations
What would happen if the same test were now applied to screen for SLE in the general population? Let us say we check all black females aged 15-44 years in New York City. This population has been studied and the prevalence of SLE in this group was determined as 80.9 per 100,000. Let us construct a similar 2 × 2 table, using the same sensitivity of 66% for a titer of ANA of 1:80 or above and a specificity of 80%. If we screened a total of 100,000 women, we would expect the following:

Table 9.3
Characteristics of a positive ANA of 1:80 or higher
Prevalence of SLE in the population tested = 80.9/100,000
Sensitivity = 66%, Specificity = 80%

		SLE *Present*	*SLE* *Absent*	
ANA titer of 1:80 or higher	*Positive*	53 (true +)	19,984 (false +)	20,037 + tests + predictive value 53/20,037 x 100 = 0.26%
	Negative	28 (false −)	79,935 (true −)	79,963 − tests − predictive value 79,935/79,963×100 = 99%
		81 SLE pts.	99,919 healthy controls	100,000 total subjects

Approximately 81 of these young women will have SLE according to our prevalence figure. Therefore, 100,000 − 81 = 99,919 is the expected number of women without the disease. Since the sensitivity is 66%, the number expected to be correctly identified as true positives is 53, and the false negative rate will be 81 – true positives (53) = 28. Since the test is 80% specific, 99,919 × 0.8 = true negatives = 79,935 and the number of false positives would be 99,919 – 79,935 = 19,984.

What has the change in prevalence from 50% to 0.08% (81 per 100,000) done to the likelihood that finding a positive ANA at a titer of 1:80 or above means presence of SLE? The positive predictive value has gone from 77% to 0.26% since only 53 among the 20,027 positives is likely to have the disease. This means that, in this population, only one of every 400 women with a positive ANA of 1:80 or higher is likely to have SLE. The other 399 individuals with a positive test are false positives.

These calculations are based on *BAYES THEOREM*, and this concept is one of the most important you can learn from our book.

WARNING #4: The *less likely* the presence of disease in the population tested, the *more likely* that an *abnormal* test result represents a *false positive*. In clinical practice, we increase the likelihood that an abnormal test in a patient represents disease by ordering the test primarily in patients with symptoms and signs suggestive of the disease. That means we are selecting a population for testing quite likely to have the disease. The prevalence of disease among these patients is likely to be as high as 20-80%. The less discriminating we are in ordering diagnostic tests, the lower the prevalence (or pre-test probability) of disease will be in the population we are testing; and, therefore, the fewer true positives we are likely to identify among those with abnormal results.

WARNING #5: *Beware* of publications that report *"predictive values"* for a test being advocated as useful. The predictive value they report is only applicable to populations with a disease prevalence *identical* to the population they tested.

In summary, principles of clinical epidemiology are fundamental to the art and science of doctoring. Keep them in mind when you are evaluating your patients.

SUGGESTED READINGS

1. Fletcher RH, Fletcher SW, Wagner EH. *Clinical Epidemiology, The Essentials,* second edition. Baltimore: Williams and Wilkins, 1988.

2. Griner, PF, Panzer RJ, Greenland P. *Clinical Diagnosis and the Laboratory: Logical Strategies for Common Medical Problems*. Chicago: Yearbook Medical Publishers, Inc., 1988.

3. Lawrence RE, Shulman LE. American Rheumatism Association. *Current Topics in Rheumatology—Epidemiology of the Rheumatic Diseases*. Proceedings of the Fourth International Conference, National Institutes of Health: New York: Gower Medical Publishing Limited, 1984.

PART II.

REGIONAL PAIN DISORDERS

Chapter 10

Approach to the Patient with a Regional Pain Syndrome

Regional pain syndromes are those conditions that present with pain limited to an anatomic area of the body like the neck, the shoulder, the hip, the low back, etc. Our approach to the patient with a regional pain complaint consists of the following steps.

EVALUATION

1. *Decide whether the pain is local or referred.* Referred pain cannot be reproduced by palpation or motion of any of the joints, ligaments, tendons, etc. of the area. In general, referred pain is more common in the upper extremities and chest than in the lower extremities.
2. If the pain is local, *establish which anatomic structure is involved* after reviewing the anatomy of the area. This will help you localize the pain to the bursae, tendons, muscles, ligaments, joints, neurovascular structures, or musculotendinous compartments. Most regional pain syndromes that have become chronic will eventually involve most of the nearby elements in the painful cycle regardless of which structure was affected first. For example, the later you see a patient with pain in the shoulder, the more likely that the patient is now suffering from deltoid bursitis, rotator cuff tendinitis, *and* bicipital tendinitis.
3. Once you have decided that the pain is originating from local structures, you should *decide whether the regional involvement is part of a systemic syndrome or not*. For example, what may originally sound like pain in the shoulder may occur in a setting of widespread or earlier achiness of other regions. In this case, the regional complaint

may actually be part of a more systemic condition like polymyalgia rheumatica, fibromyalgia, inflammatory arthritis, neuropathy, etc. Some benign conditions, like hypermobility with joint laxity, may predispose to some regional pain disorders.

4. *Assess* whether the painful condition developed in *association with acute trauma* so that a fracture or dislocation can be detected. Most isolated regional pain syndromes are associated with more chronic or repetitive trauma. This is often seen in patients who participate in competitive athletic activities, whether with others or on their own. With the current interest in health and fitness, overuse or improper use of exercise equipment may be the culprit. In these cases, we suggest patients who participate in these clubs go for more repetitions at low weights rather than fewer repetitions at higher weights.
5. *If infection is a possibility,* make certain you *exclude it*. While a history of acute swelling, heat, tenderness, redness, and limitation of motion are common in patients with a septic joint, chronic and milder presentations of infection are also seen. If any joint fluid is obtainable, feel obligated to aspirate a small amount for culture, gram stain, and to look for crystals. If enough fluid is available, a cell count and differential are also helpful. Some infections, like the syndrome of gonococcal arthritis/dermatitis, can present with monarticular, oligoarticular, or primarily a tenosynovitis picture. In these patients, culture of the involved local structure may be sterile, while culture of the cervix (in females) or urethra (in males) or posterior pharynx (in both) will confirm the diagnosis.
6. Most of the regional pain syndromes described are self-limited. Therefore, if, after a *few weeks*, a *patient has not responded* to conservative treatment with local measures, exercises, and (if necessary) local injection of steroids or lidocaine, *you must reassess the patient*. At this time, plain films or more specialized studies are indicated.

GENERAL APPROACH TO TREATMENT

Treatment is conservative and similar for most regional pain syndromes as long as conditions that may require immediate surgery or immobilization (like ligament, muscle, or tendon tears and bone fractures) or drainage and antibiotics (like infection) are excluded in every patient.

For the non-fractured, non-infected regional pain syndrome, RICE treatment is usually recommended.

R = rest
I = ice (applied for 10-15 minutes 2-3 times per day. For ease of application, a small disposable water cup filled with water can be frozen and the top third of the cup peeled off the frozen content and applied in a circular motion over the sore area.)
C = compression firm enough to give support but not so tight that ischemia or neuropathy develops.
E = elevation of the involved extremity.

In addition to RICE, partial immobilization of the area with preservation of passive and active range of motion and analgesic or nonsteroidal anti-inflammatory drugs are useful. Local injection with anesthetics with or without steroids can have excellent therapeutic results when bursitis or inflammatory arthritis is the culprit. On the other hand, injection of tendons should be avoided, especially in the athletic patient, because of the risk of tendon rupture. Narcotics are *never* indicated in the absence of fracture or tumor.

When the cause for the pain is a localized or generalized myofascial syndrome (meaning pain in tender points in muscles and tendons), low dose anti-depressants like amitriptyline or doxepin in doses of 10-25 mg qhs are very helpful. This improves restful sleep and breaks the pain/sleep deprivation/pain cycle. These drugs have not shown potential for abuse or dependence. In these low doses, anti-cholinergic side effects of orthostatic hypotension and urinary retention are quite uncommon except in the elderly.

SUGGESTED READINGS

1. Sheon RP, Moskowitz RW, Goldberg VM. *Soft Tissue Rheumatic Pain—Recognition, Management, Prevention*, second edition. Philadelphia: Lea and Febiger, 1987.

2. Hadler NM. *Medical Management of the Regional Musculoskeletal Diseases*. New York: Grune & Stratton, Inc. 1984.

3. Nakano KK. *Neurology of Musculoskeletal and Rheumatic Disorders*. Boston: Houghton-Mifflin Prof. Publishers, 1979.

4. D'Ambrosia RD, ed. *Musculoskeletal Disorders—Regional Examination and Differential Diagnosis*. Philadelphia: J. B. Lippincott Co., 1977.

Chapter 11

Shoulder Pain

A. REFERRED PAIN

Referred shoulder pain is not aggravated by shoulder motion or pressure and has characteristic features depending on the site of origin. Any process involving the *diaphragm*, which is innervated by the phrenic nerve (C_3, C_5), can refer pain to the shoulder or to the periscapular and/or supraclavicular areas. *Gallbladder inflammation or biliary obstruction* produces pain in association with meals and usually localizes to the upper quadrant of the abdomen and infrascapular area of the posterior thorax. Pain in the shoulder, upper arm, or jaw associated with exertion suggests a *coronary origin*. Acute onset of fever and shoulder pain aggravated by breathing suggests *pneumonia*, while tearing pain of the shoulder and back suggest *aortic dissection*. Constant, severe pain in the anterior neck and shoulder suggests a *Pancoast (apical lung) tumor*, which is often associated with Horner's syndrome (ptosis, miosis, anhidrosis, and enophthalmos) due to involvement of the sympathetic chain. Shoulder pain associated with paresthesias in the hand that awakens the patient from sleep is most likely due to *carpal tunnel syndrome.*

B. REGIONAL OR INTRINSIC SHOULDER PAIN

I. *Anatomy and function*

Knowledge of the gross anatomy and function of the joint provides the most help in deciding on a diagnosis (see figure 12.1). Of all the joints of the body, the shoulder has the most mobility and the least stability. It is composed of three joints: the acromioclavicular, the glenohumeral, and the sternoclavicular joints, and two gliding planes: the scapulothroacic and the subacromial planes.

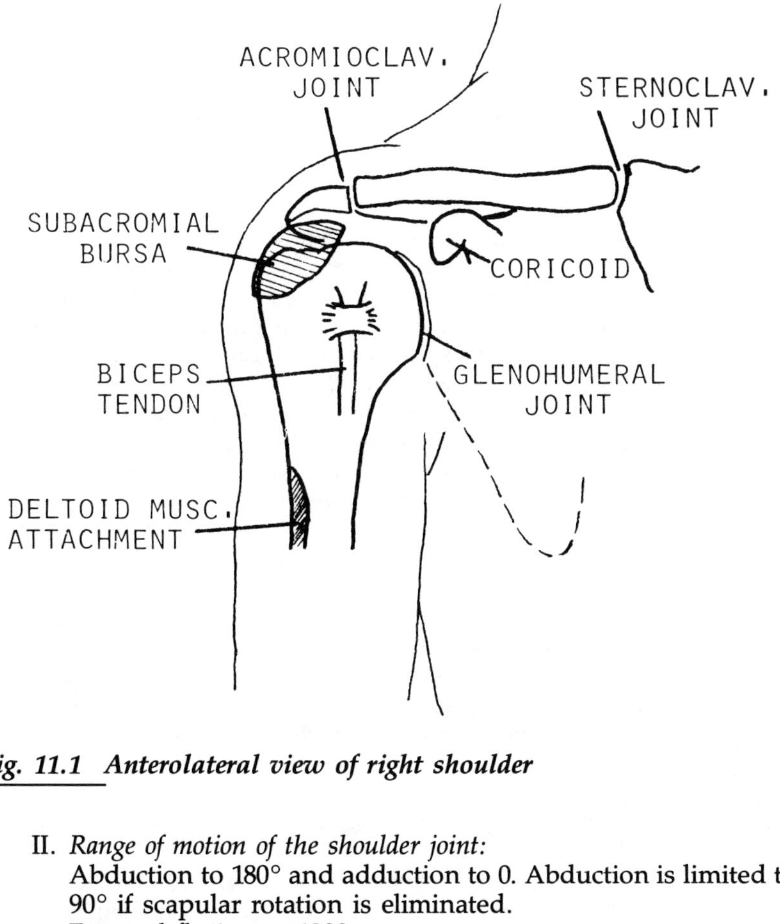

Fig. 11.1 Anterolateral view of right shoulder

II. *Range of motion of the shoulder joint:*
Abduction to 180° and adduction to 0. Abduction is limited to 90° if scapular rotation is eliminated.
Forward flexion to 180°
Backward extension to 75°
External rotation to 45-90°
Internal rotation so that the thumb of the internally rotated arm can touch the spinous processes of the thoracic spine. The specific spinous process that is reachable should be identified (i.e., T_{10}, T_{11}, etc.)

III. *Specific Syndromes of the Shoulder*

1. *Joints*

a. *Glenohumeral joint arthritis.* Crepitus on motion of the shoulder is a common finding even in normal joints, but fine crepitus with pain during motion suggests arthritis. Palpation of the superficial part of the joint capsule as it projects anteriorly just below the coracoid process produces the most pain. Isolated pain and swelling in this joint, as in any other, should be considered due to *infection* until proven otherwise. Aspiration of the joint fluid for culture and examination for crystals should be done as part of the evaluation. Any of the *inflammatory arthritides* can produce synovitis in this joint, including RA, any of the spondyloarthritides, crystal-induced arthritis, or SLE. However, isolated arthritis of one shoulder is almost never a presentation for any of these conditions, except hydroxyapatite-associated arthritis, also called *''Milwaukee shoulder,''* which is most commonly seen in elderly women. *Degenerative arthritis* is uncommon except in association with occupations that stress this joint like boxing, pneumatic hammer use, heavy manual construction work, or improper use of crutches for ambulation. *Amyloidosis* ("shoulder pad sign"), *hemochromatosis, hemophilia,* and *hemoglobinopathies* (in association with bone infarcts) are uncommon causes of arthritis with predilection for shoulder joint involvement. *Polymyalgia rheumatica,* which often presents with severe pain in the proximal musculature of the shoulder girdle, may be associated with florid synovitis and is accompanied by a high sedimentation rate (see Chapter 40).

b. *Acromioclavicular joint* arthritis is usually due to traumatic or degenerative changes. Pain occurs with *abduction* but is worse with extreme *adduction* of the arm across the chest to the opposite shoulder. Recalcitrant cases may need distal clavicle debridement and resection.

c. *Sternoclavicular joint* arthritis is very uncommon and when present is almost always septic, often in a setting of intravenous drug abuse. This joint may be involved in the spondyloarthropathies and, rarely, in gout.

2. *Bursae and tendons*
   a. *Rotator cuff tendinitis.* The rotator cuff is composed of three muscles that insert on the greater tuberosity of the humerus. Starting anteriorly, they spell SIT (supraspinatus, infraspinatus, and teres minor). A fourth rotator is the subscapularis, but it produces internal or medial rather than external or lateral rotation. Other names for this syndrome include *impingement syndrome, bursitis, calcific tendinitis,* and *shoulder periarthritis,* among others. It accounts for over 90% of the patients seen with shoulder pain. Onset of pain may be sudden or subacute. The pain is worse with abduction, and at night when the arm is dependent. There is tenderness to palpation at the point of insertion of the rotator tendons on the greater tuberosity of the humerus. Pain and tenderness are often referred distally to the deltoid insertion in the midarm. Radiographic evidence of hydroxyapatite deposits of calcium in the region of the rotator cuff is seen in 3% of normal young women and in 30% of all patients with shoulder pain. At necropsy, almost everyone over age 60 will show evidence of degeneration of the tendon fibers and 40% will show evidence of rupture.

      Physical examination maneuvers characteristic of this syndrome include the "impingement sign"—pain with forced forward elevation while keeping the scapula stable. Pain begins at 70° of abduction and disappears at 100°. In the "Codman paradox"—arm can be brought fully overhead by external rotation and abduction, or internal rotation and forward flexion, but not abduction. Rotator cuff tendinitis is most often seen in association with repetitive overhead use of the arms as occurs in many sports and occupations. It is thought to result from ischemia of the tendon during the impingement produced by hyperabduction of the arm. A treatment imperative is to keep the joint mobilized.
   b. *Subacromial or subdeltoid bursitis* usually occurs in association with rotator cuff tendinitis (see above). Some authors advocate treatment with steroids injected into the bursa as opposed to injection of the area around the insertion of the rotator cuff tendons.

c. *Bicipital tendinitis* affects the long head of the biceps tendon, which remains extrasynovial as it passes through the joint capsule from its origin in the acromion. Seen frequently in association with the impingement syndrome, it may also be seen as an isolated problem. The patient complains of pain with internal rotation, as when trying to slide the arm into a coat sleeve. *''Yergason's sign''* is often absent. The *modified Speed's sign* is more reliable. It consists of pain in the biceps tendon during resisted forward flexion of the fully supinated arm (palm up) with the elbow extended, in a position similar to that used in serving a volleyball. Rupture of this tendon may occur spontaneously and produce the *''Popeye sign,''* which is associated with minimal pain and disability. The ruptured biceps appears as a bulge.

3. *Myofascial syndromes*
   a. *Costoclavicular syndrome* presents with neck, shoulder, and arm pain in obese, heavy-breasted women with inadequate brassiere support. Improvement can be expected with long-line bras and wide shoulder straps. It may have the same pathogenesis as the military posture syndrome described under thoracic outlet syndromes below.
   b. *Myofascial Syndrome/Fibrositis/Fibromyalgia.* Defined as prominent stiffness and aching for three months or longer, with local point tenderness—"the jump" sign. In the shoulder, the rotator cuff, bicipital tendon, and the deltoid insertion sites are tender to palpation. When this pattern of tender points and stiffness is limited to the neck, shoulder and arm area, accompanied by tenderness in the rhomboids and the superior medial border of the scapula, it has been termed the *suprascapular syndrome.* The *trapezius syndrome* is similar, but the tender points are localized to the inferior medial scapular border. Treatment is the same as for generalized fibrositis (see Chapter 32).
4. *Neurovascular compression and entrapment syndromes*
   a. *Thoracic outlet syndromes* are thought to result from compression of the brachial plexus and neurovascular bun-

dle at various sites. Their validity as specific syndromes has been questioned. All are improved by changes in posture and muscle function, and surgery is unnecessary in nearly all patients.

i. "Cervical Rib Syndrome." An anomalous rib at C_7 may cause compression of the neurovascular bundle between it and the anterior scalene muscle. However, over half of individuals found to have cervical ribs are asymptomatic. *Adson's test* checks the radial pulse during a Valsalva maneuver while the neck is in maximal rotation towards the affected side and the ipsilateral arm is abducted, extended, and externally rotated. The test is positive if the pulse disappears during this maneuver. However, over 85% of normals may have a positive test, so its diagnostic usefulness is extremely limited.

ii. "Costoclavicular Syndrome" (or military posture syndrome). Compression of the neurovascular bundle between the first rib and the clavicle while bringing the shoulder down and back.

iii. "Hyperabduction Syndrome" (or pectoralis minor syndrome). Compression between the first rib and the pectoralis minor muscle during simultaneous elevation, external rotation, and hyperabduction. Symptoms occur most commonly in people who sleep with the arm in this position.

b. *Brachial Neuritis*: Pain in the brachial plexus and shoulder with subsequent weakness and atrophy of the deltoid, supraspinatus, infraspinatus, biceps, and triceps. It may be associated with a viral or post-viral syndrome. Prognosis is excellent, with slow but full recovery in over 90% within 2-3 years.

c. *Shoulder-Hand Syndrome (Reflex Neurodystrophy)*: Subacute onset of aching pain in the shoulder without localized tenderness following minor trauma, myocardial infarction, stroke, etc. It is accompanied by vasomotor instability of the hand (blanching/hyperemia), and hyperhidrosis. Early swelling evolves later into *Sudeck's atrophy* of the hand with loss of subcutaneous tissue but without becoming bound down (as would occur in scleroderma). Progressive restriction of motion and pain at the shoulder accompany progression of the syndrome. The bone scan is often diagnostic, and the process is often bilateral.

d. *Frozen shoulder/adhesive capsulitis*. This has been equated to reflex sympathetic dystrophy and to end-stage impingement syndrome. Clinical descriptions tend to vary because it is often used as a wastebasket term. Most commonly defined as a syndrome of pain and stiffness in both shoulders more common in women in the 50-70 age group, which may spontaneously recover completely in over 50% after a few months to a year. Improving the range of motion is the major goal. Sometimes, manipulation under anesthesia to "break up" the adhesions is necessary.

e. *Nerve Entrapment Syndromes*

   i. *Axillary nerve* (C_5, C_6): Entrapment occurs as the nerve exits the quadrilateral space to innervate the deltoid. It produces weakness and atrophy about the shoulder girdle. Seen in athletic individuals that perform excessive overhead activities. Radiation of the pain occurs in a sclerotomal rather than a dermatomal pattern.

   ii. *Suprascapular Nerve* (C_5, C_6): Entrapment occurs as the nerve crosses the suprascapular notch to innervate the supraspinatus and infraspinatus muscles. Produces deep pain over the upper border and body of the scapula without radiation to the arm. May lead to atrophy and weakness. Local pain is elicited on palpation of the suprascapular notch. Pain on adduction across the chest (as seen with acromio-clavicular arthritis) is typical. Also associated with excessive overhead activity in young athletic-type individuals.

   iii. *Dorsal Scapular Nerve* (C_5) may become entrapped as it passes through the fibers of the scalenus medius. This produces pain along the medial scapula with radiation to the posterior forearm and thumb and winging of the scapula.

5. *Bones*

   Osteonecrosis, leading to bone infarction close to the articular surface, can also present as glenohumeral arthritis in patients on steroids, after renal transplantation, in systemic lupus erythematosus, etc. Patients with severe destruction of the shoulder joint from osteonecrosis or inflammatory arthritis may be candidates for shoulder arthroplasty.

6. *Injuries*

   The shoulder is the most commonly dislocated joint in the body, and when dislocation occurs, the humeral head is usually displaced anteriorly. *Tears* of the glenoid labrum present with anterior shoulder pain and are becoming more common with the recent enthusiasm for throwing and racket sports. Diagnosis is established by the exposure history and arthrography.

C. EVALUATION OF PATIENTS WITH SHOULDER PAIN

Plain radiographs are helpful in excluding unusual causes like primary metastatic tumor or Paget's disease. In patients with possible trauma (whether acute or chronic), an arthrogram may be necessary to exclude a tear of the glenoid labrum, a ruptured rotator cuff, or adhesive capsulitis. Magnetic resonance imaging appears more promising than computed tomography and may eventually replace arthrography. As mentioned earlier, more specific diagnostic tests, including joint fluid aspiration and culture, EMG, and nerve conduction velocities, may be indicated. When a systemic condition is suspected, other laboratory tests may be useful.

D. TREATMENT

Prognosis is good overall for almost all of these syndromes and the treatment goals are identical. They include progressive strengthening and stretching exercises. Start with hanging the affected arm over the back of a chair while sitting, and swinging the hand around in larger and larger circles as a pendulum to mobilize the upper arm. Referral to a physical therapist, when feasible, is recommended.

Non-steroidal anti-inflammatory drugs have been shown to provide symptomatic relief. Studies have yielded contradictory results regarding efficacy of these drugs compared to local injection of steroids, but these two modalities are probably equivalent. There are no data to support combined treatment. One prospective randomized study showed improved effectiveness of steroid injection over local anesthetic alone; others have found no advantage. Injection of 40 mg of triamcinolone or methylprednisolone into the subacromial bursa, the glenohumeral joint, around the rotator cuff tendon insertion, or around the bicipital tendon, depending on your diagnosis, can be tried. Care must be exercised to inject around and not into the tendon to minimize the risk of tendon rupture. The rotator cuff may be injected through a posterior subacromial approach or anteriorly at the point of tenderness (see Chapter 6). Acupuncture is no better than placebo.

Surgery is only indicated in patients with a torn labrum or those with a destroyed glenohumeral or acromioclavicular joint. Few of the neurovascular syndromes should be treated with surgery except in unusual circumstances.

SUGGESTED READINGS

1. Cailliet R. *Shoulder Pain*, second edition. Philadelphia: F.A. Davis Co., 1981.

2. Bunker TD. Time for a new name for "frozen shoulder." Brit Med. J. 1985; 290:1233-4.

Chapter 12

Elbow Pain

A. REFERRED PAIN

Left elbow pain alone is only rarely referred from a cardiac source, in which case the pain would come on with exertion rather than with motion or palpation of the elbow. Referred elbow pain is more commonly due to disorders of the hand (like carpal tunnel syndrome) or from a shoulder or neck disorder, and this is usually obvious given the accompanying complaints. In most patients with pain in the elbow, the cause for the pain is intrinsic to the elbow.

B. REGIONAL OR INTRINSIC ELBOW PAIN

I. *Anatomy and function*

The elbow is a hinge joint formed by the olecranon of the ulna and the medial and lateral humeral condyles. The two major planes of motion are flexion and extension. In addition, the proximal and distal radio-ulnar and radio-humeral articulations allow for pronation and supination of the forearm. One of the earliest signs of disease of the elbow joint on physical examination is limitation of full extension.

Some important anatomic landmarks of the elbow include the paraolecranon grooves on either side of the olecranon process and the medial and lateral epicondyles of the humerus. The *olecranon bursa* is a large superficial bursa that overlies the olecranon and does not normally communicate with the synovial cavity. Several other bursae exist of little clinical significance. A small bursa between the distal biceps and the radial head may produce pain at the elbow during rotation of the wrist.

The *antecubital fossa* contains the biceps tendon, the radial and brachial arteries, the median and ulnar nerves, and the origin of many forearm muscles.

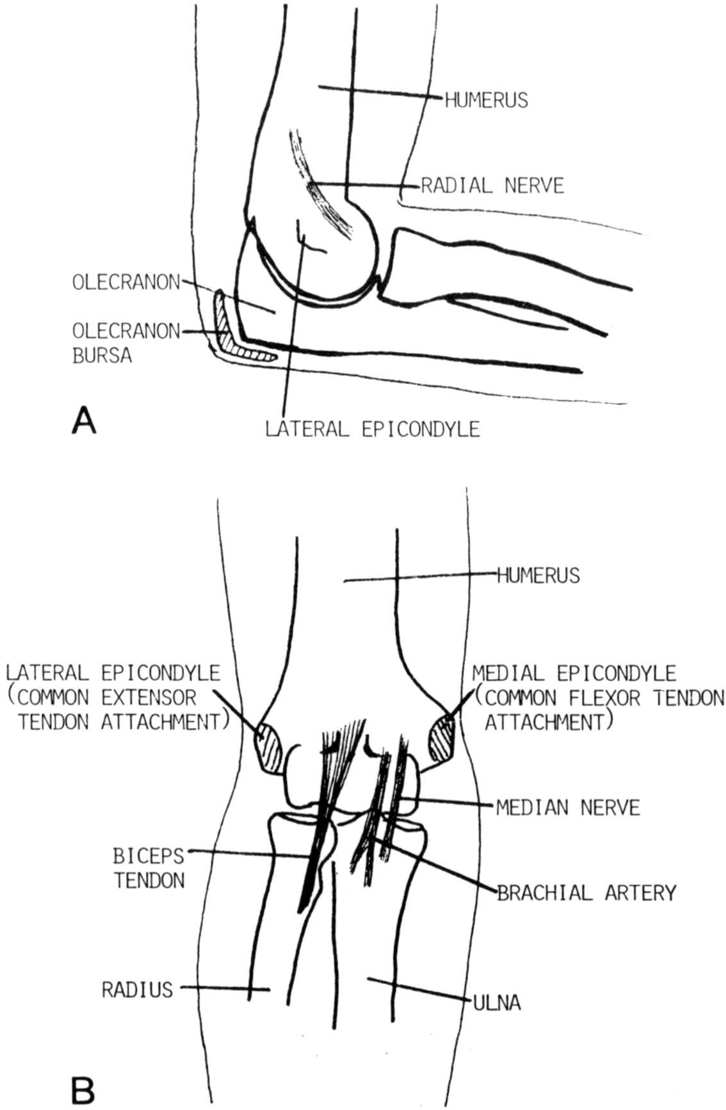

Fig. 12.1. Lateral (A) and anterior (B) views of the elbow.

The elbow should be examined with the forearm partly flexed and supported so the muscles are relaxed. You can do this by having the patient sitting across from you and resting the forearm on a table. Or you may support the patient's forearm with one of your arms while you examine the joint and adjacent areas with your other hand. *Trauma* to the elbow with impairment of the humero-ulnar joint *produces limitation* of flexion and extension only, while rotation (pronation and supination) are unaffected. When rotation is impaired, fracture of the head of the radius is usually the cause. Stabilization of the injured elbow should be in full flexion, but in general, other than immediately following trauma, elbow immobilization should be avoided.

II. *Range of motion at the elbow joint*

Flexion—Normal range is up to 150°

Extension—Should be 0° but different individuals may be able to extend 5-10° more or less. Hyperextension greater than 10° could signify presence of hypermobility, which could produce or contribute to the regional pain syndrome.

Pronation—rotating the forearm medially on the elbow joint so that the dorsum of the hand and forearm become anterior; 90° is normal.

Supination—The opposite from pronation, it consists of rotating the forearm laterally so the palm of the hand becomes anterior; 90° is normal.

III. *Specific regional syndromes*

1. *Elbow joint arthritis*

As with many other joints, arthritis of this joint must be considered *septic* until proven otherwise. The elbow is commonly involved in many of the inflammatory arthritides, in which case, involvement of other joints is usually obvious. It may also be involved in the *migratory arthritides* (for example, rheumatic fever), but again this would be clear from the history and/or physical examination. *Cysts* analogous to a Baker's cyst in the popliteal fossa may occur in the antecubital fossa. They are most likely to occur in rheumatoid arthritis, present as swelling, and dissect proximal to the fossa into the area of the triceps.

2. *Bursae*
   a. *Olecranon bursitis.* Inflammation of this readily palpable bursa is most often seen secondary to *infection* or *gout* or in association with *rheumatoid arthritis.* Aspiration of the bursal fluid for culture and cell count and examination for crystals must be done in every patient with this syndrome. If the olecranon bursitis is an isolated finding, infection or trauma is more likely. If the bursitis is due to gout or rheumatoid arthritis, a chronic draining tract may develop following aspiration. If you must aspirate to exclude an infection, you may avoid complications by using a 22-gauge or even smaller needle.
   b. *Bicipital bursitis,* from repeated trauma, as in pitching a ball, may occur in this bursa beneath the biceps tendon insertion. It presents with pain in the antecubital fossa with flexion and supination.
3. *Musculotendinous*
   a. *Lateral (or radial) epicondylitis—"tennis elbow."* This is actually most commonly seen in patients who do not play tennis but who otherwise overuse the elbow. It occurs in politicians from handshaking, also in carpenters, gardeners, dentists, etc. It presents with elbow pain at rest and during hand movement. The pain is reproduced or worsened with impeded extension at the wrist and from palpation about the lateral epicondyle. It may have an acute or chronic presentation and is most common in the 40-60 age group. In tennis players, improper holding of the racket with the elbow in front of the racket during a backhand has been denounced as etiologic. The common extensor tendon usually shows tears in this condition.
   b. *Medial epicondylitis—"golfer's elbow."* Patients present with pain in the medial condyle at the origin of the common flexor tendon. When patients present with tenderness in both the medial and lateral epicondyles, they are more likely to be suffering from fibromyalgia or a myofascial pain syndrome of the upper extremity than from isolated golfer's and tennis elbow. Look for telltale signs of these other diagnoses (see Chapter 32).

4. *Neurovascular entrapment syndromes*
   Entrapment syndromes involving the radial, median, and ulnar nerves and some of their branches have been described.
   a. *Radial nerve*:
      i. "Saturday night palsy." Wrist drop secondary to pressure neuropathy of the radial nerve either at the axilla or at the spiral groove of the humerus proximal to the elbow. It characteristically develops from falling asleep with the arm draped over a chair, usually while the patient is stuporous from too much alcohol, or from improper use of crutches.
      ii. "Radial tunnel syndrome." From compression of the nerve as it crosses the elbow posteriorly towards the lateral forearm. The pain can be reproduced by resisted extension of the third finger with the elbow extended and the forearm pronated.
      iii. "Dorsal or posterior interosseous nerve compression". Compression at the level of the supinator muscle or distal to it gives symptoms similar to "tennis elbow" or radial epicondylitis. This motor branch of the radial nerve comes off after innervation of the wrist extensors. Therefore, compression distally impairs extension of the MCPs (particularly the 5th), and thumb abduction. Extensor tendon rupture presents similarly except MCP extension can occur with the wrist flexed. Compression of the nerve occurs from tasks like hammering and carrying heavy objects.
   b. *Median nerve*:
      i. Compression of the anterior interosseous motor branch of the median nerve in the forearm may also occur and produce weakness of grip and a peculiar pinch.
      ii. the "pronator syndrome" occurs from compression of the median nerve proximal to the carpal tunnel in the belly of the pronator muscle. It produces pain during flexion of the wrist and pronation of the forearm, and paresthesias of the hand.

c. *Ulnar nerve*

i. Entrapment of the ulnar nerve in the "cubital" or elbow tunnel produces paresthesias and pain in the area of the medial epicondyle and the 4th and 5th fingers with eventual atrophy of the hypothenar and intrinsic muscles of the hand. Thickening of this or any other nerve, when accompanied by little pain, suggests a diagnosis of leprosy. Repetitive trauma from pressure on the nerve is the most common etiology.

ii. Compression of the ulnar nerve as it enters the hand through Guyon's canal (between the pisiform and hamate bones and ligament) can produce pain and numbness in the ulnar surface of the ring and little fingers. Thrombosis or aneurysm of the accompanying ulnar artery or a ganglion may be the culprit.

Treatment for all of these conditions starts by discontinuing any aggravating tasks. If symptoms persist, neuromuscular evaluation and referral is recommended.

5. *Nodules*

In the elbow, nodules are most common along the proximal extensor surface of the ulnar bone and may be due to rheumatoid arthritis, gouty tophi, xanthomas, rheumatic fever, etc. Other clues in the history and physical examination will be of help in making this diagnosis, but excision and histologic examination of the nodule provide a definitive diagnosis.

6. *Injuries*

Tears of the joint capsule or collateral ligaments are suggested by a history of trauma. In children, "nursemaid's elbow" can occur with a sudden pull of the hyperpronated forearm, leading to displacement of the radial head anteriorly.

C. EVALUATION

If the suspected syndrome is articular or periarticular, radiographs and aspiration of synovial fluid from the joint are mandatary. The synovial fluid should be cultured, the fluid examined for crystals, and a cell count and differential obtained. A peripheral white cell count and differential and sedimentation rate will also add to the history and physical examination. If a nerve entrapment syndrome is considered, nerve conduction velocities are of great help in localizing the area of pressure. Suspect bursitis when the elbow is held in extension and the olecranon bursa is boggy.

D. TREATMENT

This is usually symptomatic. For overuse syndromes, stopping, at least temporarily, whatever activity produced or aggravated the condition is useful if not absolutely necessary. Stretching exercises, learning how to use the joint, ice (or heat), and NSAIDs are helpful. Steroid injection can be beneficial but may be associated with tendon rupture and should only be considered when conservative measures fail. DMSO (dimethly sulfoxide) does not work.

For tennis or golfer's elbow, an elastic band two to three inches wide worn snugly below the elbow about one inch distal to the epicondyles may be helpful during activities that worsen the pain.

SUGGESTED READING

1. Cailliet R. *Soft Tissue Pain and Disability,* second edition. Philadelphia: F. A. Davis Co., 1988.

Chapter 13

Wrist and Hand Pain

A. REFERRED PAIN

The hand is an uncommon site for referred pain except from disorders of the cervical spine where sensory root impingement may manifest as distal upper extremity pain. Most of the pain syndromes of the wrist and hand are due to involvement of local structures.

B. REGIONAL OR INTRINSIC HAND PAIN

The hand and wrist are a finely coordinated set of bones, joints, tendons, muscles, and nerves with marvelous flexibility and strength. Anatomical features of the hand account for the overuse, entrapment, and infectious syndromes that can affect it. As with any other regional pain disorder, once the source of pain or dysfunction is identified, it becomes easier to determine whether the symptoms and findings are due to a systemic process or not.

I. *Anatomy and function*

The versatility of motion of the hand depends on its many joints and their range of motion. There is great variability in the ability of different individuals to move these joints, which accounts for some of the virtuoso performers of piano, violin, etc.

At the wrist flexion (or palmarflexion) is 90° and extension (or dorsiflexion) 70°. The degree of ulnar deviation possible is 40-50° and radial deviation 20°. Limited circumduction is possible due to rotation at the midcarpal joint. Pronation and supination do not occur at the wrist but at the proximal and distal radio-ulnar articulations.

At the metacarpal phalangeal joints (MCP), flexion is 90° and extension 30°. Variable small degrees of abduction and circumduction can also occur. At the first MCP, flexion is limited to 50°, but other movements like opposition can occur, which allows the thumb to be laid across the palm towards the little finger.

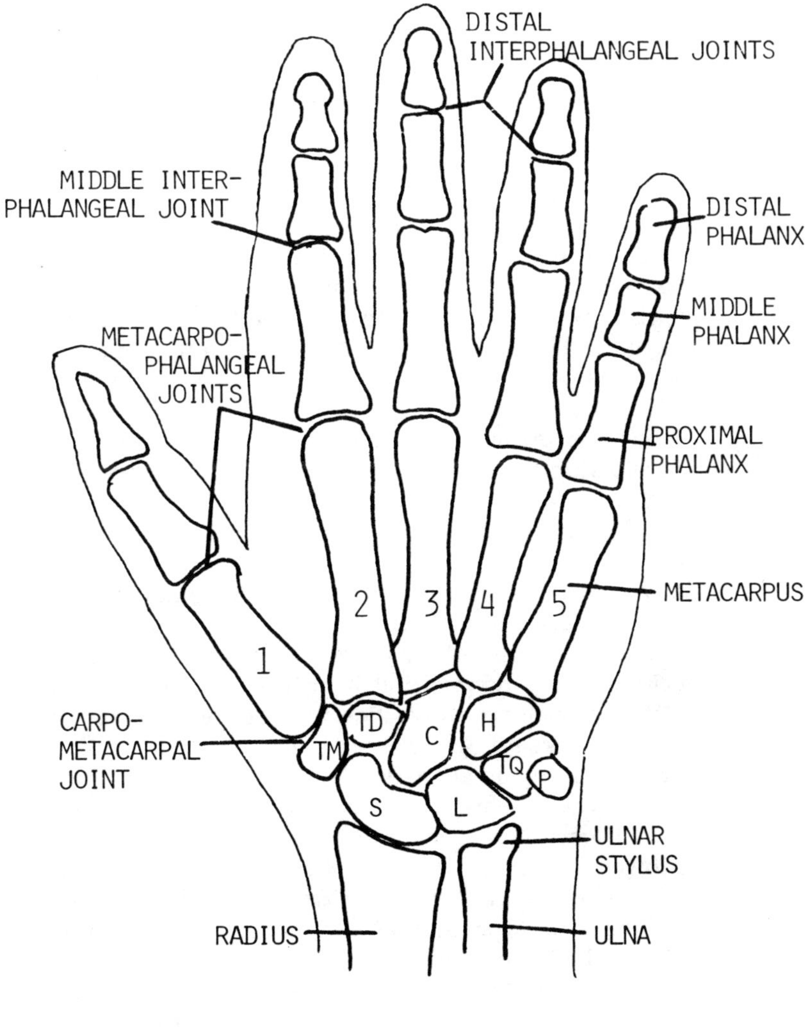

Fig. 13.1 Right dorsal hand.

Also, abduction and adduction of the thumb is possible.

The *proximal-interphalangeal (PIP)* joints can flex to 120° and extend to 0°.

The *distal interphalangeal joints (DIP)* show flexion of 80° and 0° extension.

The second through fifth flexor tendons have a common bursal ("ulnar bursa") sheath that extends from the proximal wrist into the palm. The flexor pollicis longus usually has a separate sheath.

The flexor retinaculum (or transverse carpal ligament) keeps the flexor tendons in place and forms a fibro-osseous canal—the carpal tunnel, between it and the carpal bones dorsally. The median nerve courses into the hand through this tunnel. The palmaris longus tendon crosses into the hand anterior to the retinaculum. Flexion at the wrist depends on the median (C_6, C_7) and ulnar (C_8, T_1) nerves, while extension is due to the radial nerve (C_6, C_7, C_8).

Remember during examination of the hand to look at the skin, the periungual capillaries, and the angle of the cuticle. Grip strength is greatest with the wrist extended (dorsiflexed) 30°.

II. *Specific Regional Syndromes*

1. *Joints*

Isolated arthritis of the wrist or any of the other joints of the hand, as elsewhere, must be considered infectious until proven otherwise. Many of the systemic arthritides can affect the hand. Symmetrical arthritis limited to the PIPs and DIPs, especially in association with osteophytic nodules or cysts, suggests *osteoarthritis* or *erosive osteoarthritis*. Inflammatory arthritis in an oligoarticular pattern involving the DIPs, and especially when accompanied by pitting of the nails, should suggest *psoriatic arthritis*. Predominant MCP and wrist involvement suggests *hemochromatosis*, while wrist, MCP, and PIP disease is typical of *rheumatoid arthritis*. The joint between the first metacarpal and the trapezium is the only proximal joint of the hand involved in *osteoarthritis*. It produces pain when opening doors, turning keys, etc. Eventually, subluxation and dislocation may occur at this joint with development of a "Z-collapse" thumb.

Acute onset of redness, swelling, and pain of the wrist, sometimes accompanied by fever may be due to *gout*, *pseudogout*, or *gonococcal* arthritis. If associated with periarticular calcification, it may be due to *multifocal calcific tendinitis*. Pain in the joints of the hand without arthritis may result from *"clenched fist syndrome."* Occupational reasons for similar complaints can be seen in *"writer's cramp," violinist's cramp," "typist's cramp,"* etc. Hand clenchers are often jaw clenchers as well and can present with facial pain from bruxism.

2. *Musculotendinous*
   a. Acute *tenosynovitis of the wrist* or small joints of the hands should make you consider gonococcal arthritis, RA, or gout. Other infectious and systemic conditions can also present with symptoms of tenosynovitis in the hand, but other complaints and findings usually accompany it.
   b. *De Quervain's tenosynovitis* involves the common sheath of the abductor pollicis longus and the extensor pollicis brevis. It is thought to be secondary to repetitive action or direct injury to the tendons as they come over the radial styloid. It is associated with pain in the snuffbox area during pinching motion and may have associated swelling over the radial styloid. A diagnostic maneuver is the *Finkelstein test*. The thumb is wrapped by the other four fingers against the palm. The examiner pulls the fist in an ulnar direction, stretching the painful tendons. Pain during this maneuver is considered a positive test.
   c. *Trigger thumb* is due to stenosing tenosynovitis of the flexor pollicis longus "snapping" or "triggering" and producing pain at the base of the thumb.
   d. *Trigger finger* most commonly affects the 3rd and 4th fingers in addition to the thumb. The flexor sublimus tendon locks the finger in flexion secondary to a nodule in the proximal tendon sheath.
   e. *Dupuytren's contracture* is due to nodular-like thickening of the palmar aponeurosis primarily of the 4th, 5th, and 3rd fingers in that order. It can produce a fixed flexion contracture at the MCPs and eventually the PIPs. It is most common in males (10:1 male to female distribution) and appears to be familial. By advanced age, nearly 70%

of the males in an involved family will have developed these changes. Diabetes mellitus and alcoholism, among other conditions, have been associated with this syndrome.

f. *Diabetic cheiroarthropathy* is associated with camptodactyly—a genetic flexion contracture of the PIPs. The skin over the fingers develops a waxy, shiny appearance but is not bound down as in scleroderma and is not associated with periungual changes. Other diabetes-associated syndromes are *carpal tunnel syndrome, neuropathies, trigger fingers,* and *Dupuytren's contractures.*

3. *Neurovascular syndromes.*
   a. *Raynaud's* syndrome is secondary to vasospasm. This produces two or three color changes from vasospasm (blanching-white), through prolonged stasis and desaturation (blue color), and reactive hyperemia (red). The most characteristic color is the white produced from ischemia. It may occur as an isolated cold-related phenomenon—Raynaud's disease, or secondary to any number of drugs and conditions. These include scleroderma, hypotension, trauma, frostbite, arterial obstruction, thoracic outlet syndromes, cryoproteins, use of vibratory tools (like pneumatic hammer), primary pulmonary hypertension, poisoning with lead and arsenic, pheochromocytoma and some drugs like clonidine, ergotamines, beta blockers, etc. To avoid occurrences, the whole body should be kept warm and nicotine—a potent vasoconstrictor—should be avoided. Treatment with a calcium-channel blocker may be helpful in some patients. (See Chapter 28).
   b. *Blue fingers* have been described in some women. The discoloration and pain resolves after 2-3 days. Etiology is not known.
   c. *Acrocyanosis* is a persistent cyanosis and coldness of the hands and feet associated with excessive perspiration. It is a benign condition.
   d. *Livedo reticularis* may involve the hands, the feet, and the trunk, but is most common in the feet. It produces cyanotic mottling of the skin in a fishnet appearance and

may be a manifestation of vasculitis, although it is often benign. When associated with polyarteritis nodosa, warming does not eliminate it.

e. *Reflex sympathetic dystrophy* can involve the upper or lower extremity. It produces pain in the hand and shoulder with characteristic changes of the skin and bones. It has also been called "shoulder-hand syndrome," "reflex neurodystrophy," and "post-infarctional sclerodactylia." The process is often bilateral when evaluated by bone scanning. It has been described a few weeks following myocardial infarct or stroke, or injury of the involved extremity. Sometimes it is idiopathic.

   The hand develops diffuse non-pitting or brawny edema and cyanosis. Later, the skin atrophies and appears shiny, and the muscles atrophy with the fingers held in partial flexion. Although recommended, a few weeks' course of high dose steroids is not always helpful, and the best treatment is rapid and aggressive mobilization of the limb.

4. *Entrapment syndromes of the wrist and hand*
   a. *Carpal tunnel syndrome* from compression of the median nerve as it enters the hand produces numbness, pain, and tingling of the first three fingers and half of the fourth. Motor symptoms may eventually develop. The patient gives a history of pain into the hand that wakes her up at night. Symptoms occur with any condition that stretches or squeezes the nerve—driving, writing, knitting, etc. Thenar atrophy and weakness of thumb opposition are late findings. Tapping over the nerve in the area of compression produces tingling—*Tinnel's sign*. The *Phalen test* consists of development of symptoms with acute wrist flexion against each other for one minute. Any condition that increases the volume of the soft tissues in the carpal tunnel like edema, synovitis, hypothyroidism, pregnancy, diabetes, etc. can cause it. Vitamin B_6 deficiency is associated with neuropathy rather than CTS alone.

      Surgical release should be reserved for recalcitrant cases since results are not always successful. Removable splints are available which provide excellent symptomatic relief. The recommendation is to splint at 30° of extension, which we have found may actually worsen symptoms in some patients. We prefer extension of approximately 15°. In any case, the patient should have few or no symptoms while wearing the splint. If the hand continues to hurt, the angle of the splint or the diagnosis or both may be wrong. Injection with steroids radial to the palmaris longus on the volar surface of the wrist can be helpful when the cause is inflammatory. Acute onset of bilateral carpal tunnel, especially in a young woman, is probably related to acute arthritis from rubella or human Parvovirus infection and should spontaneously resolve in a few weeks.

b. *Other neuropathies.* Injury to both the ulnar and median nerves produces the "intrinsic minus" paralytic or "claw" hand characterized by hyperextension at the MCPs and flexion at the PIPs and DIPs as well as marked atrophy of all the intrinsic hand muscles.

5. *Bones*

a. *Hypertrophic osteoarthropathy* is characterized by periosteal new bone formation at the distal metacarpals, metatarsals, and long bones. It is often associated with clubbing of the fingers and toes with loss of the nail bed angle and sponginess proximal to the base of the nails. Symptoms consist of deep burning pain in the distal extremities, aggravated by dependency and improved by elevation. On occasion, joint swelling may occur. Hypertrophic osteoarthropathy may be idiopathic, but in adults it is almost always due to lung cancer, rarely from chronic lung or liver disease. In children, congenital heart disease is most often implicated. Treatment consists of identifying the primary disorder and treating it. A similar condition may occur as part of a familial syndrome—*pachydermoperiostosis,* which begins in the teens and is inherited as an autosomal dominant with variable expression. In these patients, changes of the face accompany the changes in the hands and feet. It is a benign condition.

b. *Periosteitis* and *clubbing* may also occur from hyperthyroidism-*thyroid acropachy.* The diaphyses of the metacarpal and phalangeal bones are affected without symptoms.

c. *Avascular necrosis* may occur secondary to trauma or for no obvious reason. The most common bones affected in the hand are the lunate-*Keinbock's disease,* and the scaphoid (or navicular) *Preiser's disease. Lunate necrosis* presents with wrist pain with flexion or extension and tenderness to palpation over the lunate, which is the proximal small carpal bone that abuts the distal radio-ulnar articulation. Radiographic changes develop over a few weeks. *Navicular* or *scaphoid necrosis* presents with pain in the area of the snuff box. A similar syndrome occurs with fracture through the proximal one-third of the scaphoid with eventual avascular necrosis. Any patient with these symptoms following an injury should have repeat wrist films if the pain persists longer than two weeks.

6. *Injuries*

The most common fracture of the wrist is *Colles' fracture* in which the distal fragment of the fractured radius is displaced radially and dorsally with a resultant "dinner fork" deformity. It usually occurs from falling on the outstretched hand. *Smith's fracture* of the distal radius is the reverse of Colles'. It occurs due to a fall on the flexed wrist. Twisting injury of the metacarpals or finger bones may produce *spiral fractures. Bennett's fracture* from falling on the outstretched hand with extreme thumb abduction involves the metacarpo-trapezial joint at the base of the thumb.

Dislocations of the lunate may occur if the fall on the outstretched hand concentrates the force of the palm. *Finger sprains* are common from the finger being struck by a ball or falling on the hand with the finger in an extended position. *Gamekeeper's thumb* is due to disruption of the ulnar collateral ligament of the thumb MCP secondary to breaking rabbits' necks or, more commonly these days, while snow skiing.

7. *Miscellaneous*

Infections in the hand tend to extend according to the space involved. The most common infection is in the peringual space secondary to a hangnail. It is usually due to staphylococcus and responds to local drainage and care.

A *felon* is an infection of the pulp space of the finger. It is very painful because the volar distal finger space is limited. With progression, the infection moves along the flexor tendon sheaths. Infections in the hand may also involve the thenar or midpalmar spaces, which are separated by a fascial septum attached to the entire length of the third metacarpal. The patient can be quite ill, and open drainage and systemic antibiotics are usually required for treatment.

Tumors or nodules may occur in association with RA. *Villonodular synovitis* presents with nodules adjacent to the PIPs in women 20-30 years of age. *Xanthomas* from hyperlipidemia, *tophi* in gout, and *pseudo-rheumatoid* nodules may also occur in the hands. *Ganglia* are quite common and most often occur adjacent to the scaphoid-lunate articulation and at the radio-carpal joint. If symptomatic, they can be removed. If the diagnosis for a nodule in the hand is not obvious, it should be removed surgically for further diagnosis and treatment.

C. EVALUATION

Evaluation relies on the physical examination and radiographs when indicated (e.g., history of trauma). Aspiration of a joint may also be required. As mentioned earlier, if the pain does not resolve after a few days of symptomatic treatment and immobilization, repeat radiographs should be obtained.

D. TREATMENT

Strengthening and stretching exercises and rest are the mainstay of therapy. Inciting activities should be avoided. If the joint or tendon is inflamed but without infection, steroid injections may be useful. If splinting is needed, the hand should be in a neutral position. Fractures should be treated by orthopedists.

SUGGESTED READING

1. Sheon RP, Moskowitz RW, Goldberg VM. *Soft Tissue Rheumatic Pain*, second edition. Philadelphia: Lea & Febiger, 1987.

Chapter 14

Neck Pain

The cervical spine is a complex skeletal structure containing seven cervical vertebrae, 26 separate joints, including the 14 apophyseal joints and the 12 joints of Luschka, and five intervertebral discs. The bones and joints plus other structures in the neck such as ligaments, tendons, nerves, and vessels can all produce pain. To complicate matters further, pain can be referred to the neck from remote organs, and structures in the neck can refer pain away from the neck. Neck pain and stiffness is a very common problem, occurring in at least half of working people.

A. REFERRED PAIN

Pain originating in distant visceral or somatic organs can be referred to the neck, shoulder, arm, or the pectoral girdle region because these organs still retain the same cervical root innervation from embryologic development. In contrast to pain developing from a local inflammatory process, areas of referred pain are not tender to palpation and have no associated muscle spasm, although hyperesthesia may be present. Often there may be associated nausea, vomiting, or cramping. The visceral organs most often responsible for referred pain to the neck and pectoral region include: heart and coronary arteries, the apex of the lungs, aorta, diaphragm, temporomandibular joints, pancreas, esophagus, or gallbladder.

B. REGIONAL OR INTRINSIC PAIN

The pain-sensitive structures in the neck are the vertebral bodies, intervertebral discs, apophyseal (or facet) joints and uncovertebral joints (or joints of Luschka), vertebral arteries, cervical spinal cord, dura, motor and sensory nerve roots, and ligaments, tendons, and muscles.

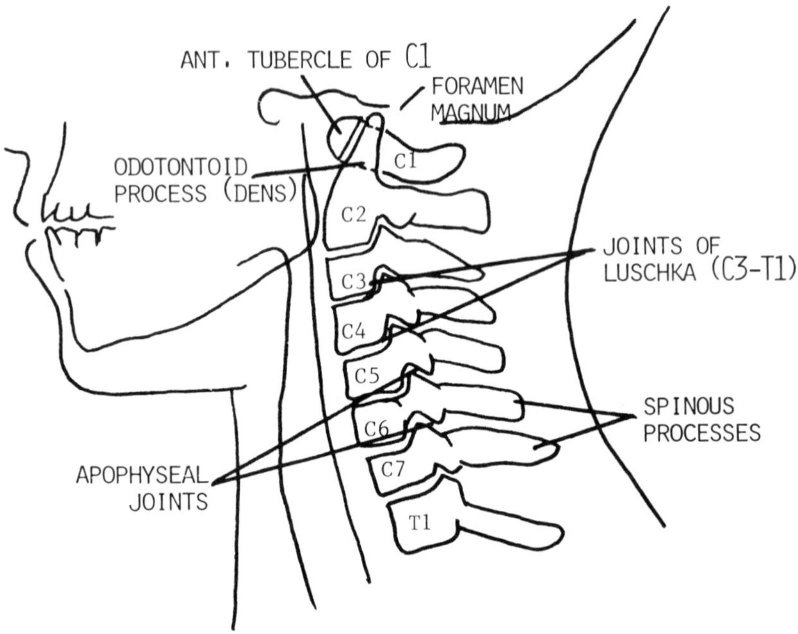

Fig. 14.1 Lateral view of cervical spine.

I. *Anatomy and Function*

The neck has as its main function support of the head. This is achieved via two very specialized vertebrae, the atlas and axis, and by ligaments, muscles, and capsular structures. Other important functions performed by the neck are movement of the head and neck, support of the shoulder girdle, and support of the thoracic inlet.

The greatest degree of motion of the head occurs between C_1 (the atlas) and C_2 (the axis). Rotation of the head of 90° to either side occurs at this level. Range of motion of the rest of the cervical spine consists of 30° lateral bending, 45° of forward flexion, and 30° backward extension. During flexion of the neck, the intervertebral foramina are more open than during backward extension. Similarly, during lateral bending, the diameter of the foramina decreases on the bent side. The most mobile part of the cervical spine is the C_4, C_5, C_6 segment, which is also at greatest risk of degenerative changes.

II. *Specific Regional Syndromes*

1. *Joints*

Inflammatory or degenerative changes of the apophyseal or uncovertebral joints usually causes localized pain. Inflamed synovial tissue, especially at the uncovertebral joints in patients with RA, can erode into bone and soft tissues. Synovial destructive changes also occur commonly at C_1-C_2 with destruction of the odontoid process of C_2 and loss of the transverse ligament of the atlas (C_1), which normally holds the odontoid in place. If the disease progresses enough, the odontoid may migrate proximally into the foramen magnum and can cause compression of the medulla. This presents with intermittent quadriparesis, without sensory loss, and neck pain. If untreated, sudden death is a major risk. Subluxation may also occur at other levels of the cervical spine, (e.g., C_4 on C_5 occurs often in RA patients with long-standing disease). The resultant instability noted with flexion can produce subluxation and myelopathy.

Fusion of inflamed facet joints can occur in spondyloarthropathies such as ankylosing spondylitis and result in a fixed spine with no motion possible. The facet joints are also involved commonly by degenerative arthritis, resulting in loss of articular cartilage, decreased motion, and pain, and in some may lead to cervical spinal stenosis discussed below.

2. *Musculotendinous*

a. *Myofascial pain.* Muscular aching can occur either from a local injury, from strain (overuse), or as part of a systemic illness. Most commonly local neck pain occurs from holding the head in an awkward position (often flexed while working at a desk) for too long a period of time. The strain of supporting the heavy head against gravity accounts for tensing the posterior cervical-occipital muscles.

A very common neck injury occurring in automobile accidents is "*whiplash.*" Pain resulting from this type of injury is primarily ligamentous and muscular. Systemic illnesses can also cause pain and/or weakness such as polymyositis, polymyalgia rheumatica, and fibromyalgia. A careful history and examination, together with the results of pertinent laboratory data (e.g., sedimentation rate and muscle enzymes), will allow the correct diagnosis to be made.

b. *Acquired torticollis* ("wry neck") results from a painful spasm of the sternocleidomastoid muscle on the affected side secondary to trauma, or from an acute upper respiratory viral infection (usually seen in children). It tends to be self-limited and treatment should be conservative till it resolves in a few weeks. *Spasmodic torticollis* is a focal dystonia of adults that presents more commonly in women than men with involuntary turning of the head to one side which progresses from occurring intermittently to eventually becoming continuous. Treatment consists of biofeedback and, in severe cases, denervative surgical procedures.

3. *Neurovascular and entrapment syndromes*

Disease of the intervertebral discs and spurs of the vertebral bodies may cause nerve root impingement. This can result in both neck pain and pain referred to the shoulder and arm. Depending upon which nerve root is irritated, pain may be perceived in the shoulder, arm, hand, or head. Understanding dermatomal distributions of the various nerve roots will simplify the search for the level of nerve root entrapment. The Spurling maneuver is helpful in eliciting if the pain is radicular or not by applying pressure to the head while the patient is seated with the head rotated towards the bad side and tilted down. Pain in the shoulder during this maneuver is a positive test for impingement. Cervical root impingement syndromes are more often due to osteophytes at the foramina than to disc protrusion and tend to be chronic. Acute onset of radicular symptoms is more suggestive of disc protrusion. The symptoms associated with specific nerve roots are outlined below.

C_5—shoulder and upper arm pain and decreased biceps reflex

C_6—pain in the radial aspect of the forearm with paresthesias in the thumb and diminished biceps and brachioradialis reflexes

C_7—dorsal forearm pain and paresthesias of the index and middle fingers with decreased triceps reflex
C_8—ulnar forearm pain and paresthesias of the ring and little fingers with diminished triceps reflex

Cervical spinal stenosis leads to spinal cord compression and produces two types of pain: dermatomal (or neurologic) and sclerotomal (or myalgic). Sclerotomal pain is experienced as dull, muscle ache type pain with superimposed electric lancinating pain. Dermatomal pain produces paresthesias and a sensory level of radicular symptoms. Bowel and bladder dysfunction may be present and are useful physical findings to establish this diagnosis. However, some patients with cervical spinal stenosis and myelopathy may present with little else besides an inability to walk accompanied by upper motor neuron signs in the lower extremities (increased reflexes, clonus, extensor Babinski response) and lower motor neuron signs in the upper extremities (diminished reflexes, atrophy and fasciculations).

Lateral plain films of the cervical spine are helpful in screening for spinal stenosis. The canal, measured from the posterior aspect of the vertebral bodies to the end of the lamina (where the spinous process begins) should be greater than 13-15 mm. A congenitally narrowed or abnormally shaped spinal canal and the long term result of degenerative arthritis of the facet and uncovertebral joints with its attendant osteophytes encroaching further on the canal are the most common cause. Treatment consists of surgical decompression.

4. *Injuries*

The vertebral bodies can be sources of severe pain if fractured or invaded by tumor or infection. Physical examination would show focal tenderness to palpation of the involved bony structures and associated muscle spasm. In these cases, care must be exercised when moving the spine to prevent injury to the cord. The presence of fever, chills, and cutaneous or other primary infection would suggest vertebral or disc infection as the source of neck pain.

C. EVALUATION

To evaluate neck pain of local origin, an assessment of the local anatomy is essential. The bony anatomy can be visualized quite easily with radiographs done in the posterior-anterior and lateral projections. Oblique views should be obtained if one is looking for nerve root entrapment as the neural foramina are well visualized on this view. If instability of the spine is in question, views of the neck both in flexion and extension are required. Careful review of the neck films should be made, looking for bony destructive lesions, subluxation at any level, neuroforaminal narrowing, disc space narrowing, osteophytes, and degenerative changes.

Other radiographic techniques are also available to address specific anatomic abnormalities found on plain films or suspected by history and physical examination. A CT scan with (or without) a cervical myelogram, or magnetic resonance imaging (MRI) study of the cervical spine can detect abnormalities of the spinal cord and nerve roots. If a radicular problem is being considered, nerve conduction studies and electromyography (EMG) may be useful.

Lastly, if irritation or infection of the meninges is felt to be a strong consideration as a source of neck pain, examination of cerebrospinal fluid (CSF) is essential. The lumbar puncture can usually be performed with ease, and opening and closing pressures should be measured and fluid sent for the appropriate studies, including cell count, Gram's stain, culture, glucose, protein, etc. Blood tests pertinent to evaluation of neck pain include Westergren sedimentation rate, muscle enzymes, and a chemistry panel with close attention paid to the calcium, phosphorus, and alkaline phosphatase levels.

D. TREATMENT

For general maintenance of neck motion and function, range of motion exercises are encouraged. These include moving the head in forward flexion, extension, lateral flexion, and rotating the chin to look over each shoulder. They are often best performed when under a hot shower, taking advantage of the relaxing quality of heat. These exercises are particularly useful to maintain motion in patients who have local musculoligamentous problems or in patients with inflammatory joint disease.

Intermittent cervical traction has been used to treat pain from radiculopathies with variable results. If enough force is used, traction can actually separate the articular surfaces of the zygapophyseal joints, which may relieve nerve root compression and irritation. Traction is also used to reduce the inflammatory response and muscle spasm and to improve the circulatory status within the epidural spaces of the spinal cord and nerve roots. Traction can be done either in the supine or seated position. It is usually done intermittently for 10-20 minutes, beginning with 8-10 pounds and gradually increasing it to about 20-30 pounds to get enough force to produce alignment and relax the muscles. Cervical collars are indicated when you want to limit spinal motion to reduce pain and muscle spasm or to maintain alignment and support the musculoskeletal structures when they are inadequate (e.g., fractures of vertebral bodies). The collar can be soft and provide little support (soft, foam rubber collar) or rigid with fixation to the skull (Halo vest), used primarily in patients who have sustained cervical trauma (vertebral fractures, subluxations, etc.) or undergone cervical spine surgery.

Aspirin or nonsteroidal anti-inflammatory drugs are useful for pain relief for musculoligamentous or joint pain but will not relieve spinal cord or nerve root entrapment syndromes. If muscle spasm is a major component of the pain, Flexeril 10 mg qhs is helpful. Surgery is resorted to *only* if conservative medical management has failed in the treatment of radiculopathies or if there is evidence of myelopathy, fracture, or instability.

SUGGESTED READINGS

1. Bland JH. *Disorders of the Cervical Spine*. Philadelphia: W.B. Saunders, 1987.

2. Cailliet R. *Neck and Arm Pain*, second edition. Philadelphia: F.A. Davis Co., 1981.

Chapter 15

Chest Wall Pain

A. REFERRED CHEST PAIN

The etiology of chest pain in any one patient may be serious intrathoracic or intra-abdominal disease or a benign myofascial pain syndrome. Unlike other regional pain disorders in which referred pain from remote or internal organs is unlikely, *chest pain is often referred*. Patients with this complaint must be evaluated carefully to exclude internal organ involvement before making a diagnosis of a local pain disorder. The history and physical examination are the most useful tools in making this determination.

Sensory impulses from deep structures in the chest and upper abdomen that are innervated by the first six thoracic roots (T_1-T_6) may be referred to the chest—so-called "six dermatome band" and produce deep retrosternal or precordial pain. The characteristics of the pain are helpful in suggesting the likely source. On the other hand, the severity of the pain bears little relationship to the severity of the condition. The precipitating and relieving factors, the location, quality, timing and severity are all useful in making a diagnosis. In instances when the pain has several overlapping characteristics, more than one condition may be present, as occurs in *''linked angina''* in which esophageal reflux may produce a cardiac ischemic response. Remember, presence of a local cause for the pain does not exclude a more serious condition being present.

Anginal or ischemic cardiac pain is usually referred to the retrosternal area rather than the precordium or left inframammary area. The neck, jaw, shoulder, or medial left elbow may also be sites of referral. It is typically associated with exertion and relieved by rest. The cause for ischemia may be narrowing of the epicardial coronary arteries, increased oxygen demand by the myocardium, or diminished blood and oxygen supply from any cause. Therefore, *aortic stenosis,*

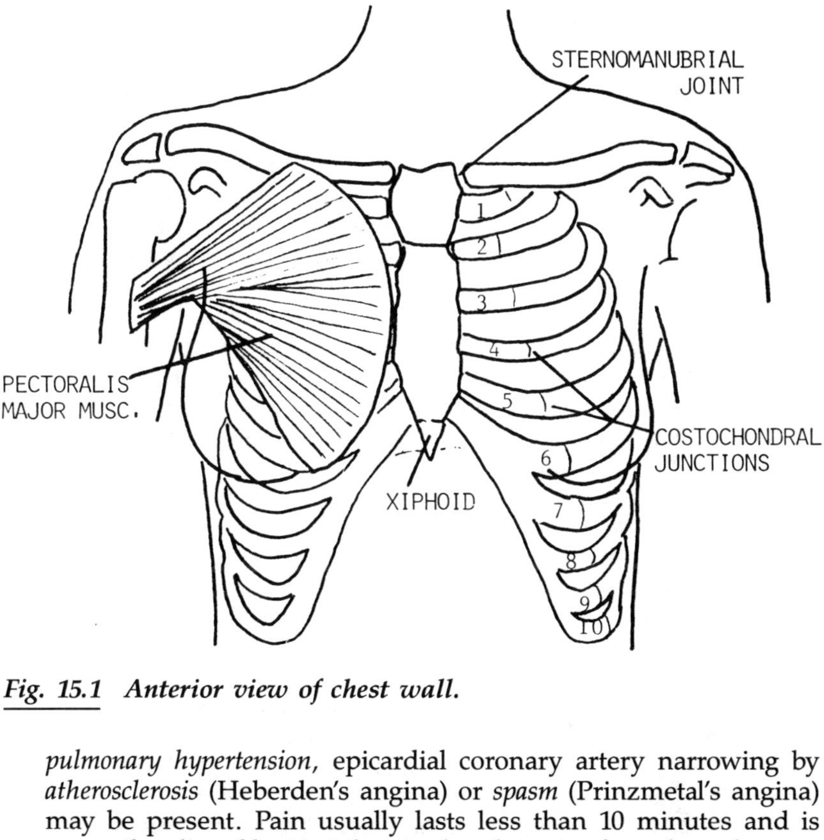

Fig. 15.1 Anterior view of chest wall.

pulmonary hypertension, epicardial coronary artery narrowing by *atherosclerosis* (Heberden's angina) or *spasm* (Prinzmetal's angina) may be present. Pain usually lasts less than 10 minutes and is promptly relieved by nitroglycerin, but the pain of esophageal spasm may also respond to this treatment. Angina pain is described as a substernal pressure or squeezing discomfort associated with shortness of breath rather than a stabbing, short-lasting pain. In addition to exertion in general, minor exertion on cold days, onset soon after a heavy meal, and emotional upset are also recognized precipitating factors. In some populations, an exercise test looking for electrocardiographic changes of ischemia may help establish the diagnosis. At other times, cardiac catheterization is necessary. As a general rule, the stress test is likely to produce false positive findings in patients with a low likelihood of disease (like premenopausal women). Among patients with a high probability of coronary disease (e.g., middle-aged men), an abnormal test is usually a true positive.

Aortic dissection pain is usually sudden in onset and described as a very severe "tearing" pain that radiates through to the back. It is seen in patients with a history of systolic hypertension, and is often accompanied by asymmetric upper extremity and cervical arterial pulses and the diastolic blowing murmur of aortic valvular regurgitation. A radiograph of the chest usually shows a widely dilated aorta.

"Cardiac" non-anginal pain may occur in association with mitral valve prolapse, "panic attacks," and in chronic smokers. In some of these patients, a cause for the pain other than a myofascial chest wall syndrome is not found. How "cardiac" is the etiology of the pain is unclear, and each individual patient must be carefully evaluated.

Diaphragmatic pain is pleuritic in nature—that is, intensified by breathing, coughing, or laughing. When the central diaphragm is involved, the pain may be referred to the superior border of the trapezius muscle and the supraclavicular fossa.

Esophageal reflux and/or spasm may be felt deep in the thorax or in the epigastrium and typically occurs when lying down or bending over, when the likelihood of reflux is greatest. Unpredictable spasm of the esophagus as seen in *"nutcracker esophagus"* produces similar pain and is diagnosed by esophageal manometry. Rupture of the esophagus during vomiting (*Boerhaave's syndrome*) occurs suddenly and produces extreme dyspnea.

Gallbladder pain from inflammatory and/or obstructive disease most commonly occurs after meals and eventually localizes to the right upper quadrant. When obstruction is present, icterus (elevation in the bilirubin) and elevated alkaline phosphatase accompany the syndrome. When complicated by infection, systemic signs of fever and leukocytosis are present.

Gas entrapment syndromes from aerophagia and trapped swallowed air in the gastric fundus or in the splenic flexure producing distension of a viscus (stomach or colon) can be perceived as very severe by the patient. It is most often seen in anxious individuals.

Hiatal hernia (diaphragmatic hernia) is very common but almost always asymptomatic. Very rare complications include strangulation of a herniated portion of the stomach through the diaphragmatic hiatus. When pain is present, esophageal reflux is the most common cause.

Mediastinal pain is uncommon even with a large tumor present in the mediastinum. When present, the pain is pleuritic and substernal and unrelated to exertion, meals, or motion. Mediastinal emphysema, if acute, can produce pain.

Myocardial infarction is the diagnosis most feared by the patient presenting with chest pain and by the physician doing the evaluation. It is similar to anginal pain and felt as a midsternal tightness or pressure. It is unrelieved by nitroglycerin, lasts more than 30 minutes and is often accompanied by nausea, sweating, pallor, and shortness of breath. Vomiting, arrhythmias, and shock may also occur, and the diagnosis is confirmed by elevated myocardial enzymes in the patient's serum and by characteristic evolution of the electrocardiogram. A ventricular or atrial gallop is almost always present.

Pancreatitis/pancreatic pseudocyst and pancreatic cancer may be associated with "boring" pain in the epigastrium that goes through to the back. Other history and findings usually point to the cause of pain.

Peptic ulcer disease of the stomach or duodenum may refer pain to the epigastrium but its characteristic relief with food helps to differentiate it from other causes.

Pericardial pain is unrelated to meals, exertion, or motion but is worse when lying supine and better with the patient sitting up and leaning forward. A pericardial rub is often heard, but it may be muffled when a large effusion is present. The ECG may show characteristic changes, and definitive findings by echocardiography help confirm the condition.

Pleural pain is well-localized and timed to coincide with respiratory motion. When due to a fractured rib or pneumonia, pleural pain is often accompanied by involuntary splinting of the respiratory muscles on the involved side. It is worsened by breathing, coughing, and laughing and is described as knife-like. A pleural rub is usually present.

Pneumonia/pneumonitis produces pain when the process involves the pleural or diaphragmatic surfaces. It is pleuritic (meaning associated with breathing) and may improve when accompanied by pleural fluid.

Pulmonary embolism may produce varying degrees and types of pain depending on the consequences. When accompanied by *pulmonary infarction*, it will behave like the pain from pneumonia. Dyspnea, hemoptysis, and bronchospasm may accompany the pain. When the embolism is massive, shock, cyanosis, and death may supervene. While simultaneous ventilation perfusion lung scans showing non-matched segmental defects are suggestive, a definitive diagnosis requires a pulmonary angiogram.

B. REGIONAL OR INTRINSIC CAUSES OF CHEST WALL PAIN

I. *Anatomy and function*

The chest expands during inspiration, thanks to the primary muscles of respiration—the diaphragm and intercostal muscles. This necessitates normal motion at the sternoclavicular, costoclavicular, and costovertebral joints. To ascertain the degree of chest motion, chest expansion at full inspiration and again at full expiration are important. Measurement is usually made at the level of the nipple and is useful to follow disease activity in the spondyloarthritides. Normal chest expansion should be 5-6 cm or more.

II. Specific syndromes of chest wall structures

1. *Joints*

a. The *costochondral (costosternal)* junctions may become painful and produce chronic intermittent chest pain reproduced by palpation of one or more of these joints. It is a common finding in patients with fibromyalgia. *Costochondritis* with pain and inflammation of these joints is characteristic of some of the spondyloarthritides. When limited to the second or third costochondral joint and associated with swelling, it is called *Tietze's syndrome.*

b. *Rib tip or slipping cartilage syndrome*—Pain from this syndrome is described as "stabbing" and is reproduced by palpation of the rib cage with the "hooking maneuver." This is done by holding the edge of the rib cage at the 8th-10th ribs anteriorly and gently pulling anteriorly.

c. *xiphoidalgia*—diagnosed by finding tenderness of the xiphoid process. It is a cause for chronic retrosternal pain. It is thought to be due to arthritis at the xiphisternal junction.

d. *Sternoclavicular hyperostosis* is a syndrome of unknown

etiology recently described in the U.S. but well recognized in Japan. There is pain and swelling of the sternoclavicular joint with bony erosions of the clavicle and hyperostosis of the sternum. Palmo-plantar pustulosis is an associated finding. Treatment is symptomatic and nonspecific.

2. *Musculotendinous*
   a. *Sternalis syndrome* is a myofascial syndrome characterized by pain and tenderness of the sternalis muscle overlying the sternum.
   b. The *intercostal muscles* may be involved by viral infection, as in *epidemic pleurodynia*, also known as "Bornholm's disease" or "the Devil's grip." The pain is intermittent and very severe when it occurs. The illness usually lasts a few days and has been associated with infection with each of the following viruses: coxsackie B, coxsackie A, and ECHO.
   c. The *pectoralis major syndrome*. This muscle may become painful and develop tender points. Often this syndrome occurs as a part of generalized fibromyalgia or as a more limited myofascial syndrome.
3. *Neurovascular and spinal syndromes*
   a. *Herpes zoster pain* ("shingles") is a burning, itching pain in a dermatomal distribution due to infection of the spinal root by the varicella-zoster virus. The telltale vesicular rash usually develops within a few days. It is always unilateral and does not cross the midline. In some patients, the pain persists after resolution of the rash, producing "post-herpetic neuralgia," which may be quite difficult to treat. Topical application of irritants like Ben-Gay may be helpful.
   b. *Thoracoabdominal radiculopathy*—While it originates from the thoracic nerve roots in the spine, this condition may present with chest or abdominal pain, sensory polyneuropathy, and weight loss. It is most common in diabetics but may be seen in non-diabetics. The diagnosis is made by electromyography (EMG) of the thoracic paraspinal muscles which show fibrillation potentials and positive sharp waves indicative of active denervation of

the muscles. However, remember *EMG changes of denervation* take up to *three weeks* to show up. The pain is often described as "vise-like," severe, and constant. Typically it is worse in the evening and nonpleuritic in nature. Often it reaches a peak in a few weeks and eventually resolves after a few months.

c. *Herniated intervertebral thoracic disc* is quite uncommon and represents less than 1% of patients with surgical disc disease. However, it does occur and may produce intermittent or constant back pain with radicular extension. When long-standing, it may press on the cord sufficiently to present with numbness and weakness of the lower extremities, bilateral spastic paralysis, and urinary retention. Surgical decompression does not always reverse the neurologic deficit. It is diagnosed by CT scanning and myelography or MRI.

4. *Bones*
   a. *Rib fracture*—produces local pleuritic pain. The fracture site can be identified by careful palpation of the painful area and confirmed by radiographs, or a bone scan.
   b. *Periosteitis* can occur in association with osteomyelitis or bruising and bleeding into the periosteum.
   c. *Expansion of the bone marrow by tumor or normal marrow* is usually asymptomatic unless there is involvement of the periosteum or a pathologic fracture.
   d. *Osteomalacia* due to vitamin D deficiency from any cause is associated with bony tenderness and aching of bones.
5. *Breasts*

   Pain in the breast may rarely be due to a malignant or benign tumor but is more commonly associated with fibrocystic disease, infectious mastitis, or abscess. If there is any doubt abut the diagnosis or if the patient is over age 40 or has a family history of breast cancer, a mammogram is indicated.

C. EVALUATION

Begins with a careful history and physical examination. Other studies are done as indicated but should include a chest radiograph and an electrocardiogram if there is any suspicion of pleuropulmonary or cardiac disease. More specific testing to diagnose some of the conditions that produce referred pain may be needed in individual patients.

D. TREATMENT

This varies depending on the condition found. For more specific recommendations for the non-rheumatic causes of pain, the reader is referred to an internal medicine text. For the local pain syndromes, immobilization of a fractured rib, use of low dose amitriptyline for myofascial pain syndromes and non-steroidal anti-inflammatory drugs (NSAIDs) for patients with arthritis or for analgesia is sufficient.

SUGGESTED READINGS

1. Semble EL, Wise CM. Chest pain: A rheumatologist's perspective. Southern Med J. 1988; 81:64-88.

2. Sellman MS, Mayer RF. Thoracoabdominal radiculopathy. Southern Med J. 1988; 81:199-201.

Chapter 16

Low Back Pain

Symptoms of low back pain inconvenience about 100% of the population at some time in their life and account for a large proportion of lost work days and disability. Unfortunately, we are not able to pinpoint precisely what structure is responsible for the pain in a majority of patients. Most of the literature approaches low back pain through a temporal classification as acute (lasting less than six weeks), subacute (between 6-12 weeks), and chronic (over 12 weeks), and any of these episodes may recur. Assuming there is nothing to suggest infection or bony trauma, most patients with low back pain improve within a few days to a few weeks, although recurrences are common.

If active disc herniation with spinal nerve root impingement is found, surgery may be indicated. As with other regional pains, our job is to make sure the cause for the pain is not something that requires specific treatment—like infection, bleed, tumor, etc. If the syndrome is associated with bowel and bladder abnormalities, suspect a *cauda equina syndrome*.

A. REFERRED PAIN

Most of the causes of low back pain are local to the lumbosacral spine and related structures; however, intra-abdominal and retroperitoneal processes may present with back pain. In patients over age 50 presenting with acute low back pain, a *ruptured abdominal aneurysm* must be considered. These patients' pain usually has a very acute onset and is not associated with motion. Femoral pulses (one or both) may be diminished. An emergency ultrasound often can establish the presence of the aneurysm. In a patient on anticoagulants, even in the absence of any history of trauma, a *retroperitoneal bleed* must be ruled out.

Pyelonephritis or *renal colic* should always be evaluated and ruled out with a urinalysis in patients presenting with acute low back pain. Occasionally *lower lobe pneumonia* with pleural involvement may produce pain felt in the mid-back, but the pleuritic component and other findings easily identify its correct origin. *Pancreatic disease*—either a pseudocyst or pancreatitis, may also present with posterior high lumbar pain, but again other associated findings are helpful in pointing to the pancreas as the source.

In males, acute and chronic *prostatitis* may present as low back discomfort. A rectal examination and examination of the urine are usually diagnostic.

Finally, almost any acute or subacute septic process may be accompanied by *non-specific back* pain, for example, bacterial endocarditis. This is probably related to the myalgias associated with the release of lymphokines involved in the inflammatory response. Other musculoskeletal structures, like the hip and knee joints, can sometimes refer pain to the low back because of changes in gait and posture, but this is not common. However, true leg length discrepancies of over 1 cm should be corrected by a shoe lift.

B. REGIONAL OR LOCAL PAIN

I. *Anatomy and Function*

The low back is comprised of the five lumbar vertebrae, the sacrum, the coccyx, and the iliac bones. Many powerful muscles originate from and insert into these bony structures and distally into the femur. Several bursae of clinical importance are present in these areas, some of which are discussed later (see Chapter 17 on hip pain). Finally, all of the lower nerve roots and the lumbar, sacral, and pudendal plexi arise from the lumbosacral area. The spinal cord ends at the level of L_1, and the rest of the spinal canal down to the coccyx is filled by the cauda equina and filum terminale. The anatomy of the back is such that it provides stability and strength to the body and allows for several motions.

Extension (or backward extension) is produced by contraction of the erector spinae (or sacrospinalis), which is a composite of several muscles with intricate relationships with the vertebrae. Normal extension is 20-30°. *Lateral bending* is normally 30-35°, and *lateral rotation* with the pelvis fixed by the examiner is 30-35° to either side. *Forward flexion* normally produces a change in the normal lumbosacral lordosis so that the curve of

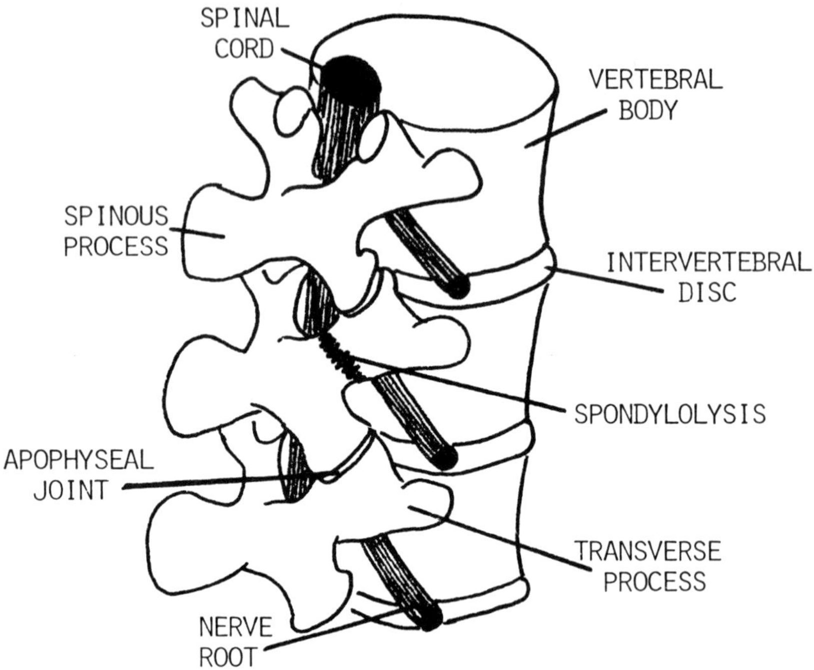

Fig. 16.1. Posterior oblique view of spine.

the back is reversed during bending. Loss of the ability to reverse this lordosis is common in patients with musculoskeletal low back pain. Mobility during forward flexion is limited in spondylitis and is measured by the Schober test. Forward flexion is accomplished by the muscles that originate from the anterior surface of the vertebrae like both psoas (major and minor) and the quadratus lumborum. The spinal column can flex as a whole 90°. The abdominal musculature accounts for about 30% of forward flexion motion.

The sacroiliac joints have an articular capsule and synovial membrane, and the joint is widest in an AP diameter at the lower end of the joint. Strong ligaments hold the two sides of the joint in place. The vertebrae articulate with each other through the intervertebral disc, composed of a soft nucleus pulposus encircled by the resilient annulus fibrosus with its strong Sharpey fibers at the periphery. In addition, the lumbar vertebrae articulate with each other and with the 12th thoracic vertebra cranially and the sacrum caudally through the facet or apophyseal joints. These are diarthrodial joints between the inferior articular process of one vertebrae and the superior process of the one below. There are ligaments that attach between the anterior aspects of each vertebrae (the dense anterior longitudinal ligament), and the posterior aspects of the vetebral bodies anterior to the spinal cord (the posterior longitudinal ligament). The posterior ligament is less strong than the anterior one, which may explain why posterior herniation of the nucleus pulposus is more likely to occur than anterior herniation. In addition, the ligamentum flavum goes between the laminae of adjacent vertebrae, and the transverse and spinous processes attach to each other through the supraspinous and interspinous ligaments.

C. EXAMINATION

The complete screening physical examination should be performed (see Chapter 3) and, at the least, the pelvic, rectal, and abdominal areas examined, in addition to the neuromuscular, vascular, and joint examination outlined here. When examining the rectum, make note of sphincter tone (should be present), tenderness of the prostate, tenderness of the pyriformis muscle and coccyx, and any masses. Observe the patient walk, look for antalgic gait, scoliosis, and other abnormalities. Scoliosis that is seen only while the patient is standing is functional, while scoliosis that remains when the patient is bending forward is structural. Tilting the trunk to one side suggests paravertebral muscle spasm.

Ask the patient to walk on his heels towards you so you can see the distance from the floor to the raised toes. Drooping of the toes on one side suggests weakness of the anterior leg muscles that dorsiflex the foot and possible L_5 root impingement. Then ask the patient to walk away from you on his toes. A drooping ankle suggests weak gastro-soleus muscles, possibly related to S_1 root impingement. Now measure for the Schober test. With the patient standing, draw a mark over the spine at the level of the iliac crests and make two more marks, one 10 cm above this level and the other 5 cm below. Then ask the patient to try touching the floor by forward flexion, and measure the distance between the upper and lower marks. The distance normally goes from 15 cm to 20 cm. The finger to floor test—measuring the distance from the tip of the fingers to the floor with the patient bending forward—is affected by tightness of the hamstrings and is not as good a measure of posterior spinal distraction. Less than 5 cm lengthening of the lumbosacral spine during forward flexion suggests spondylitis.

Next have the patient rotate his trunk while you hold the pelvis fixed with your hands on the iliac crests. Palpate the spine carefully looking for bony abnormalities, such as a step off in the lumbar spine from spondylolisthesis, increased warmth (as in a septic osteomyelitis or discitis), and paravertebral spasm or tenderness. Check the back for tender points—which are located at the gluteal origins of the iliac crest, over the episacral fat pads in the area of the SI joints. Palpate the sacroiliac joint itself and other tender points at the sciatic notches and ischiogluteal bursa, the trochanteric bursa, in the hamstrings (proximal to their insertion), the popliteal fossae, the gastrosoleus muscles, the fibular heads, and the fasciae lata.

With the patient lying supine, measure true leg length from the anterior superior iliac spines to the medial malleoli. Normally, there is no more than 1 cm difference. Straight leg raising beginning with the uninvolved side is done now with the patient supine. Normally, there should be no back discomfort on flexing the leg at the hip with the knee extended, but in some patients with a herniated disc, pain in the ipsilateral leg and buttock may occur soon after the hip is flexed. Acute dorsiflexion of the ankle of this leg by the examiner also produces worsening pain because it produces stretching of the nerve root, conversely, flexing the knee relaxes the pull on the retroperitoneal structures and relieves this pain. Sometimes pain in the bad side is felt during the straight leg raising (SLR) examination of the opposite side—so called "crossed SLR." Unfortunately, neither of these tests is sufficiently sensitive or specific to be diagnostic.

SI joint disease is associated with pain on compression of both iliac crests simultaneously as can be achieved with the patient in a lateral decubitus position, by pressing the iliac crest on top against the side lying on the examination table. If there is any suggestion of muscle atrophy, bilateral leg and thigh circumference should be measured. The strength of each muscle group, the presence or absence of fasciculations, and the deep tendon reflexes should be checked. An absent or diminished knee jerk is found with compression of the L_4 root, while a decreased ankle jerk suggests S_1 compression. To test L_5, the strength of the dorsiflexors of the big toe are tested. Light touch and proprioception should be checked to evaluate the sensory nerves and spinal afferents. Finally, the arterial pulses of the leg need to be checked—femoral, popliteal, dorsalis pedis, and posterior tibial arteries.

II. *Specific Syndromes*

1. *Joints*

   a. *facet joints*. Arthritis in these joints is most commonly due to *osteoarthritis* and is quite common, with almost everyone showing some degenerative changes by age 60 or above. Symptoms are pain, decreased range of motion, and in some cases, nerve root compression. It has been shown that facet arthritis may produce "sciatica" pain without nerve root entrapment. If facilities are available, injection under fluoroscopy of a local anesthetic into or around the facet joint may be followed by complete resolution of the pain. The levels of the lumbar spine most frequently affected are the L_4, L_5 and L_5, S_1 levels. This is probably one of the most common causes for chronic or recurrent low back pain. Rheumatoid arthritis does not affect the facet joints of the lumbar spine, and neither do gout or pseudogout although there are occasional case reports. *Charcot neuroarthropathy,* a late sequelae of neurosphylis, may involve the spine. The radiographic findings of marked disorganization of the joint and the abnormal neurologic examination help establish the diagnosis.

   b. *sacroiliac joints*. These joints are characteristically involved in the *seronegative spondyloarthropathies* (ankylosing spondylitis, psoriatic spondylitis, Reiter's syndrome, and gut-associated spondylitis). The clinical picture is quite characteristic, including insidious onset at a young age, stiffness worse in the morning but improving with exercise and a chronic course. In women, sacroiliitis appears to be less associated with symptoms and needs to be distinguished from *osteitis condensans ilii*. This sclerotic process involves primarily the inferior portion of the ilium without erosions or bridging ankylosis to the sacrum. It has little clinical significance.

In the spondyloarthropathies, the SI joint is one of the first involved and shows extensive sclerosis on both sides (ileum and sacrum) with pseudowidening, cysts, erosions, and eventual ankylosis. On examination, there is pain over the SI joints and limitation of motion. Other findings include involvement of the spine with extensive ligamentous and enthesis calcification. Treatment is more specific and aimed at directing eventual ankylosis to occur in a functional position (see Chapter 35).

Other systemic arthropathies only rarely involve this joint, and degenerative changes are usually limited to the inferior aspect of the joint with sclerosis but without erosions or ankylosis. Infection of this joint is uncommon except in intravenous drug abusers, in whom gram negative organisms are also common. Ankylosing and bowel-associated spondylitis tend to be symmetrical and, in addition to loss of the SI joints, show typical marginal discrete syndesmophytes at the periphery of the vertebral bodies. In contrast, Reiter's syndrome and psoriatic spondylitis often involve one SI joint to a greater extent than the other and are associated with asymmetric and exuberant calcification at the enthesis, so called non-marginal syndesmophytes.

c. *disc degeneration* or *intervertebral osteochondrosis* develops as the disc ages. The nucleous pulposus becomes dessicated and friable, and crevices develop within the disc ("vacuum phenomenon") seen on plain films. As the process continues, there is loss of disc height and herniation of the disc into the vertebral body (Schmorl's or cartilaginous nodes) with reactive sclerosis of the vertebral margins. Men are more commonly affected, and the condition increases in prevalence with age. *Infection* of this area (discitis) shows similar changes except the sclerotic margins are ill-defined and there is an associated soft tissue mass. Infection usually results from spread of osteomyelitis. Certain organisms are more likely to affect the spine, including staphylococcus and *Mycobacterium tuberculosis*. Less common but distinctive syndromes can be seen with *Brucella* and *Salmonella*.

d. *Spondylosis deformans* or spinal osteophytosis is similar, but the degenerative process of the disc is most prominent at the periphery of the annulus (where strong Sharpey's fibers attach to the vertebral rim). Disruption is followed by disc extrusion anterior and lateral. This process is worst if the nucleus pulposus has not lost tissue turgor and the individual is very active. The response to these stresses is new bone formation—osteophytes. This condition is also very common. By age 50, as many as 60% of women and 80% of men have developed these changes. Heavy labor may predispose to their development. Neurovascular impingement is rare since most of the displacement and reactive osteophytes are anterior.

   Calcification of the intervertebral disc may occur in AS and is also seen in alkaptonuria (ochronosis), pseudogout, hemochromatosis, hyperparathyroidism, acromegaly, amyloidosis, poliomyelitis, and prior surgery. H vertebrae or "fish mouth" vertebrae are typical of *sickle cell disease* due to compression of the osteoporotic vertebral bodies by a normal intervertebral disc.

e. *degenerative spondylolisthesis* is an acquired abnormality of vertebral alignment secondary to degenerative changes in the spine, primarily due to osteoarthritis of the facet joints. As the apophyseal joints sclerose and narrow, the tight fit between the superior and inferior facets is lost and the superior vertebral body can slip forward over the inferior vertebra. This slipping forward is called spondylolisthesis. As with facet joint arthritis, the most commonly involved level is L_4, L_5 and is more common in older women. When the changes are such that the superior vertebra slips backwards, it is called retrolisthesis. Retrolisthesis is more common in the upper lumbar area of L_1, L_2. The degree of slip can vary, but it commonly involves a quarter of the vertebral body (Grade I). Symptoms vary from none, to low back pain with some degree of nerve root compression, to severe spinal claudication as seen in spinal stenosis.

2. *Musculotendinous and ligamentous syndromes*
   a. *''Mechanical'' low back pain* is a term applied to acute onset during some activity of low back pain which is self-limited and related to the activity. This pain tends to recur and is often associated with abnormal discs and facet joint arthritis (see above). It is a poorly defined wastebasket term for pain that cannot be ascribed to a specific entity but which lacks the tender points of myofascial back pain and the radicular component of sciatica (see below).
   b. *Enthesopathies.* Seronegative spondyloarthropathies are characterized by calcification at the sites of ligament and tendon insertion.
   c. *Myofascial pain* is a more chronic low back pain syndrome characterized by tender points in the low back and leg described in the physical examination above (also see Chapter 3). The pain is constant but varies with the weather. Treatment with exercise, massage, heat, and, if needed, for poor sleep with low dose antidepressants are all helpful.
   d. *DISH—diffuse idiopathic skeletal hyperostosis* is associated with extensive ossification of the anterior and lateral ligaments. The diagnosis is made from the plain films showing "dripping wax candle" appearance of the calcified ligaments in four contiguous vertebrae. These patients have been thought of as mostly asymptomatic. However, in some studies, stiffness of the thoracolumbar area, limitations of spinal motion, and involvement of more peripheral joints by the excessive calcification of ligaments have been reported. Treatment is symptomatic. These patients are prone to develop spinal stenosis (central or peripheral).
   e. *Pyriformis syndrome* may be due to spasm of the pyriformis muscle which occupies the greater sciatic foramen or to compression of the sciatic nerve as it exits from underneath the muscle itself. It presents with low back/buttock pain, worse after prolonged sitting, and tenderness on palpation of the sciatic notch and the lateral rectal wall.

Injection of the muscle with an anesthetic and steroid mixture provides relief.

3. *Neurovascular and entrapment syndromes*
   a. *Sciatica* is the term used to describe low back pain with associated radicular symptoms of neuritic pain that radiates into the leg. It often has an acute onset and is thought to be due to posterior disc herniation pressing on the spinal nerve root. Herniation occurs in over 90% of patients at the L_5 root, the S_1 root or both. Rarely the L_4 root is involved. As reviewed earlier in the physical examination section, L_5 root (L_4, L_5 disc) involvement radiates to the SI joint, the hip and the lateral thigh and leg. There is weakness of dorsiflexion of the big toe. An S_1 root (L_5, S_1 disc) herniation presents with similar pain but with more involvement of the heel and the fifth toe. The ankle jerk is decreased. The pain of sciatica is worsened by maneuvers that increase intraspinal pressure like coughing, sitting, and Valsalva maneuver, and is relieved by lying down on the side with flexed hips and knees.

      A midline posterior disc herniation can produce a *cauda equina syndrome* similar to that seen with an intraspinal tumor with low back and perineal pain, bowel and bladder incontinence, and weakness of the legs. This is an emergency that should be evaluated immediately with a CT scan and surgical consultation.
   b. *Epidural (or extradural) pressure,* usually from metastatic tumor (most commonly breast, prostate, lung, lymphoma, or myeloma), presents with low back pain. The pain is worse when the patient is lying down at night and is better when the patient is standing. Radicular features may be present (like worse pain with coughing and sneezing). Weakness eventually develops, with paraparesis and a sensory level and bowel and bladder symptoms. When a diagnosis is made from plain films and/or CT, oral steroids and local radiation provide prompt relief of symptoms. Transverse myelopathy similar to this can develop acutely from an epidural abscess or hemorrhage.

4. *Bones*

   The lumbar spine is a common site for congenital anomalies. The most common in asymptomatic adults is a failure of fusion of the vertebral arches leading to *spina bifida*. *Paget's* disease of bone may involve the spine, and *metastatic tumor* to the vertebrae (as opposed to the epidural space) is most commonly seen as a lytic lesion of a pedicle.

5. *Injuries*

   Trauma to the lumbar spine can range from ligamentous and muscle sprain to unstable fracture. Since acute severe trauma cases are seen by emergency room physicians, the patients we are more likely to see are those with less ominous injuries. *Compression fractures* in patients with osteopenia, particularly those with a history of steroid use, are very common even in the absence of significant trauma. They are usually stable because of intact spinal ligaments. Fractures of a *transverse process*, a *spinous process* or the *lamina* may be missed initially at the time of the trauma and may present a few days later with persistent local pain.

6. *Other Syndromes*

   a. *Failed back syndrome* is the term applied to patients with previous back surgery for possible herniated disc who fail to improve following surgery. There are two major reasons for this syndrome. One is inappropriate selection of patients for surgery. Such patients are likely to have suffered from a myofascial syndrome without true herniation as a cause for the pain. The other cause of persistent or recurrent symptoms is post-operative inflammation and/or fibrosis such as arachnoiditis. With the recent advent of microsurgery and the marked improvement in diagnostic tests, we should see fewer and fewer of these patients.

   b. *Polymyalgia rheumatica.* Although more likely to involve the upper extremities first, patients may present with pain and stiffness of the low back and pelvic girdle. However, the likely spread to involve the shoulder girdle and the elevated sedimentation rate in an elderly person suggest the diagnosis.

D. EVALUATION

Plain radiographs are usually unnecessary in most patients who are otherwise healthy who present with acute low back pain. Circumstances in which lumbar spine films are likely to be useful include patients with a history of significant trauma and patients over age 50. In addition, findings at the time of the visit such as fever, elevated ESR, neuromotor deficits, history of weight loss, suspicion of spondylitis, prior steroid use, drug or alcohol abuse, known previous malignancy, and pending litigation or compensation are good reasons for plain films. An AP and lateral pelvis is usually sufficient. Although not 100% sensitive, sacroiliitis is usually detectable in the patient with long-standing inflammatory pain. Finally, every patient who does not respond to a few weeks of conservative treatment should be evaluated with spine films.

CT scanning with or without myelography and MRI are state of the art techniques for evaluating the patient further once plain films have been obtained. Plain radiographs suffice to exclude fractures, tumor, sacroiliitis, spondylitis, and infection, but disc herniation is only visible with CT or MRI. Bone scan should be ordered if there is a high probability of malignancy or fracture which is undetected on plain films. A major problems with the interpretation of abnormal findings in scans and films is their lack of specificity. Many totally asymptomatic individuals have various abnormalities or degenerative changes found when films or scans are done for an unrelated reason. Therefore, finding these changes in symptomatic patients will not necessarily explain the symptoms. In a study of magnetic resonance imaging (MRI) of asymptomatic women, there was a linear increase in the prevalence of disc degeneration with age so that by age 70, nearly 100% of those examined had degenerated discs detected by MRI.

As mentioned earlier, a urinalysis should be done if there is even a remote possibility of renal infection or stone. In patients with fever, a complete peripheral blood count and differential and other studies as needed should also be obtained.

E. TREATMENT

Bed rest "with bathroom and dining privileges" helps. The optimal time period is not known, but recent data from patients with acute low back pain, show that two days of bed rest provide the same functional outcome as seven days, with much less time lost from work.

There are *no* indications for narcotics in low back pain from *any* cause except tumor. There are no data to prove that oral or parenteral steroids help improve outcome or shorten pain and disability despite anecdotal enthusiasm for them.

The traditional laminectomy is rarely done now, and probably caused as much (and oftentimes *more*) pain than it relieved. With the newer techniques involving microdiskectomies, disruption of ligaments, tendons, muscles, and bone is almost nil, yet the obtrusive herniated disc can be removed. This can be done as outpatient surgery, and the patient walks away from the hospital with little more than a 1" circular bandaid.

Chemonucleolysis by injecting chymopapain into the troublesome disc enjoyed a brief revival, but experience with it has been disappointing and it is no longer used.

Posture, work, and hobbies need to be modified to suit the patient. Sitting for too long or not being able to sit at all are conditions associated with back pain, and so are lack of satisfaction in the job and level of stress. The amount of pressure on the spine increases with sitting, walking, coughing, and jumping. Lifting a heavy object also increases this pressure several fold, with the highest load occurring during lifting with the knees straight rather than bent. Although the Williams flexion exercises to strengthen the abdominal muscles are excellent in asymptomatic patients, they should not be done in patients with back pain, especially if a herniated disc is likely. Isometric exercises of the abdominal and pelvic areas are better.

SUGGESTED READINGS

1. Frymoyer JW. Back pain and sciatica. N Engl J Med. 1988; 318:291-300.

2. Deyo RA, Diehl AK. Lumbar spine films in primary care: Current use and effects of selective ordering criteria. J Gen Intern Med. 1986; 1:20-25.

Chapter 17

Hip Pain

A. REFERRED PAIN

Pain from the thoracic and lumbar spine may be referred to the hip and buttock. Likewise, disease of retroperitoneal structures, like a psoas abscess, may also refer pain to the hip. More often, hip pain is due to local causes and progresses from pain mostly on walking and standing, to pain with motion even while lying, to pain at rest. Hip joint pain is felt in the groin and buttock and is referred to the knee. Abnormalities of any nearby structures may resemble hip and groin pain, including fractures of the pubis and ischium, right- or left-sided colonic or pelvic disease, and inflammation or swelling of any of the vessels or structures around the area. A complete hip examination includes an abdominal, rectal, and genital examination.

Observing the patient walk and having him stand on one leg at a time also helps assess the degree of hip joint involvement. A patient with hip joint disease walks with an *antalgic or painful gait,* characterized by avoidance of weight bearing on the painful side. When there is weakness of the abductors, as may occur with poliomyelitis, the patient tilts toward the good side while standing, but tilts toward the weak side while walking, producing a *Trendelenburg* or *abductor limp.*

B. SPECIFIC REGIONAL SYNDROMES OF THE HIP

I. *Anatomy and Function*

The hip joint is a weight-bearing joint composed of the femoral head and the acetabulum. The acetabulum is formed by three pelvic bones—the ischium, the pubis, and the ilium. The acetabulum forms an incomplete ring which is completed in its lower portion by a very strong transverse acetabular ligament which stretches between the posterior and anterior aspects of the inferior acetabulum. A complete ring of fibro-

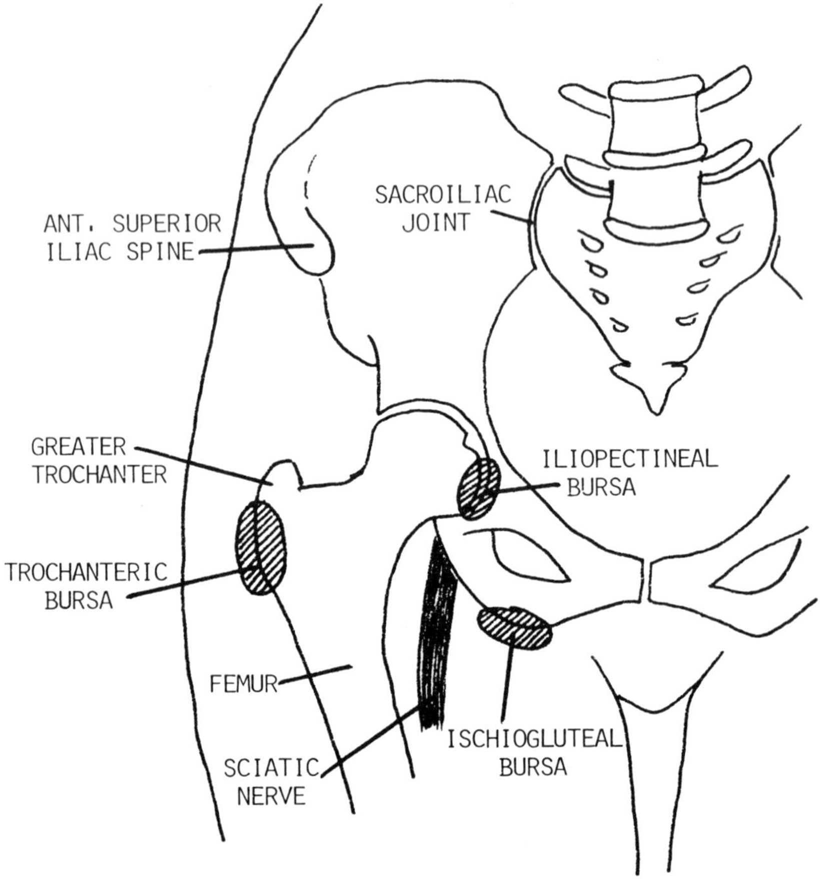

Fig. 17.1. Anterior view of hip and pelvis.

cartilage—the labrum—is found covering the acetabulum, and the femoral head is stabilized against it by a very tough fibrous joint capsule that extends from the bony rim of the acetabulum to the femoral neck. This structural arrangement provides for a very stable joint with remarkable range of motion. A small ligament carries the blood supply to the femoral head from the center of the acetabulum—the ligamentum teres.

II. *Range of motion*—(quite variable from individual to individual but should be the same in both sides for each person).

flexion of 120°—150° and extension to 15°
adduction to 25-30° and abduction of 20° to 45°
internal (or medial rotation) about 30° and external (or lateral) rotation about 45°.

FABERE test (same as Patrick's test or heel to knee test) tests for *F*lexion, *A*bduction, *E*xternal *R*otation and *E*xtension. It is done by having the patient place her foot on the knee opposite the painful hip while abducting, flexing and externally rotating the bad hip and flexing the knee. The examiner then pushes on the bent knee. Hip or SI joint disease may be associated with pain during this maneuver. However, it can only be done and interpreted in the absence of pathology of the knee. True leg length is measured from the anterior superior iliac spine to the medial malleolus. Leg length discrepancies up to 1 cm are considered normal and not a cause for hip or back pain.

III. *Specific Regional disorders*

1. *Joints*

   Arthritis of the hip joint is most commonly degenerative. It often presents with a limp. It occurs more frequently in men than in women and tends to be unilateral. Congenital or acquired childhood hip defects have been identified as a cause for the arthritis in about 40%. Among these defects are:

   a. *Legg-Calvé-Perthes disease*—avascular necrosis of the proximal femoral epiphysis. Occurs mostly in boys between the ages of 4 and 8 years.
   b. *slipped capital femoral epiphysis* usually presents in the teen years but may show up later.
   c. *congenital hip dysplasia* is an abnormality of the acetabulum where there is insufficient coverage or depth for the femoral head; occurs more commonly in women and may present early or late in life.

   While hip arthritis is most often degenerative, it may be (and often is) involved by any of the inflammatory arthritides. As with any other joint, isolated hip pain must be considered septic until proven otherwise, particularly if the patient is febrile or has an elevated peripheral white count and/or a "left shift."

2. *Bursae*

   There are multiple bursae in and around the hip joint, three of them can become inflamed and produce characteristic pain in the ipsilateral hip, groin, or buttock.

   a. *trochanteric bursa* is between the iliotibial band and the greater trochanter and is easily identified by eliciting pressure pain over the greater trochanter. It produces night pain and tenderness that is located approximately two inches posterior and superior to the trochanter. Hip motion is normal except for guarding during internal and external rotation and resisted flexion.
   b. *ileopectineal bursa* is between the iliopsoas muscle and the anterior hip joint and communicates with the joint in approximately 15% of individuals. Pain is localized to the area of the groin lateral to the femoral artery.
   c. *ischiogluteal bursa* covers the ischial tuberosity and may be a source of pain. Inflammation of this bursa has been called "weaver's bottom."

3. *Musculotendinous structures*

   a. *ileotibial band contraction*. This band is part of the fascia lata and extends from the pelvic bones (ileum) over the greater trochanter and lateral thigh to insert into the lateral tibia and the head of the fibula. When contraction of this band is severe, the affected leg is shortened because of flexion contracture of the knee and accompanying flexion, abduction, and external rotation of the hip. Knee instability is a commonly associated problem. Several tests have been advocated to prove abnormal contraction of this band by stressing the leg in abduction (*Ober test*) or in adduction (*modified Thomas test*). Sprain of this band occurs in dancers and athletes. Symptoms are similar to trochanteric bursitis, but there is pain on passive adduction of the hip only.

      A *"snapping hip"* may be associated with a taut ileotibial band. It is a painless noise caused by the band moving over the greater tuberosity of the femur. Treatment for a contracted iliotibial band consists of local injection with steroids (do not exceed 50-60 mg of Aristospan or Depo-Medrol) and stretching exercises. These are done with the patient lying on the good side by the edge of a bed or table and flexing and adducting the tight leg at the hip so that the band stretches down as the leg falls towards the floor. Weights can be added to the ankle of the tight leg while doing this to exert greater gravitational pull on the band.

When a "snapping hip" causes pain, in addition to the iliotibial band, other musculotendinous structures may be the cause, including the psoas muscle, the adductor tendons, and tears of the labrum. Pinpointing the cause may be quite difficult.

b. *Fascia lata fasciitis* is a myofascial syndrome with similar symptoms as above. It may lead to eventual contraction and tightness of the fascia lata as described above. Treatment is the same.

4. *Neurovascular and entrapment syndromes*
   a. *Reflex neurodystrophy.* This poorly understood condition more commonly affects the upper extremity. When it affects the lower extremity, the hip may be involved but the foot and ankle are more commonly affected. There are changes in the skin which becomes taut and shiny, and in the bones, which develop patchy osteoporosis. "Causalgic" pain, as this type of pain is described, is worse on weight-bearing and is the usual presenting complaint. It may occur following trauma, stroke, etc. Treatment consists mainly of early mobilization.
   b. *Charcot neuro-arthropathy.* The hip may be affected in patients with neuropathy and myelopathy from tabes dorsalis. Characteristic findings are a large joint effusion and relatively little pain. Radiologic findings include resorption and fragmentation of the articulating surfaces, severe disorganization of the joint, and osseous hypertrophy. Treatment is symptomatic, but some bracing may be necessary to maintain ambulation.
   c. *Obturator nerve entrapment* may occur from a hernia through the obturator canal. The nerve supplies the adductors of the hip. Pain and paresthesias in the groin

and proximal inner thigh are characteristic. It is confirmed by relief of symptoms with a local nerve block. Rarely, the herniated loop of bowel may strangulate and produce intestinal obstruction.

d. *Meralgia paresthetica* is a common neuropathy involving the lateral femoral cutaneous nerve as it passes through the inguinal ligament and the sartorius muscle and then exits through the fascia lata. The most common causes are local pressure from rapid weight gain, pregnancy, prolonged sitting with the legs crossed, etc. It is a benign self-limited disorder.

5. *Bones*

a. *Paget's disease* of the hip joint usually produces pain. Radiographs are diagnostic, and serum alkaline phosphatase is usually increased. Treatment consists of NSAIDs, and, if the pain is not controlled, diphosphonates or calcitonin.

b. *Ischemic necrosis* of bone can be seen in association with systemic steroids, trauma, sickle cell disease, chronic renal disease, SLE, etc. It is usually bilateral, but one side may be more symptomatic than the other. Eventually it requires replacement of the hip, although when diagnosed early, core decompression and/or bone grafting of the femoral head may be therapeutic.

c. *Osteomalacia* is associated with "pseudo-fractures" that are painful and tend to occur in the pubic rami and the proximal femur. They are actual fractures that respond to vitamin D replacement therapy.

d. *Metastatic cancer* in the hip joint bones can be the source of pain. A radiograph is usually sufficient for diagnosis. Occasionally, a bone scan or CT scan is necessary. It usually presents in patients with known cancer of the breast, prostate, or lung. Other cancers are less commonly involved. Remember that multiple myeloma involvement of the skeleton is associated with lytic lesions on plain radiographs and negative bone scans.

6. *Injuries*

Injuries of the hip joint are a major problem in the elderly, many of whom are osteopenic and suffer from some degree of impairment in multiple sensory organs. This makes them particularly susceptible to falling with consequent hip fracture. Because of the common comorbidity with multiple other illnesses, mortality from hip fracture is in the range of 25-50%. A patient with probable osteopenia (because of age or other risk factors) and hip pain should be *presumed to have a fracture* even in the face of negative radiographs, since a hairline fracture may not become obvious until there is some callus formation. If you are in doubt, a bone scan will reveal the area of bony injury.

C. EVALUATION

The history and physical examination (including abdomen, genitalia, and rectal areas) are important and may be supplemented by radiographs or scans looking for joint or bony abnormalities.

D. TREATMENT

This totally depends on the conditions found. Resting the joint by use of crutches or use of a cane in the hand opposite the bad leg can help with ambulation. Exercises emphasize achieving the full range of motion while supine. Weight-bearing is delayed in cases of fracture or tumor. Bursitis and tendinitis are treated with local or systemic anti-inflammatory drug therapy.

In some cases, surgery is indicated. Total hip replacement has achieved remarkable technical advances and is truly one of the more miraculous rehabilitative surgeries available. In the hands of a good surgeon with a competent anesthesia and medicine staff, it has minimal morbidity and mortality risks. Rheumatologic, orthopedic, neurologic, or oncologic consultation should be requested as appropriate.

SUGGESTED READING

1. Cailliet R. *Soft Tissue Pain and Disability,* second edition. Philadelphia: FA Davis Co. 1988.

Chapter 18

Knee Pain

A. REFERRED KNEE PAIN

Knee pain may be referred from hip disease or lumbosacral nerve root impingement, but in general, most knee pain originates from local structures.

B. REGIONAL OR INTRINSIC KNEE PAIN

I. *Anatomy and Function*

The knee is the largest joint of the body. It has three compartments with a common synovial cavity. These are the *medial* and *lateral* joint spaces between the distal femur and the proximal tibia, and the *retropatellar* compartment between the patella and the femoral groove. It is stabilized by the powerful tendon of the quadriceps femoris which encases the patella and inserts on the tibial tuberosity. This tendon is shared by four muscles—the vastus medialis, the vastus intermedius, the vastus lateralis, and the rectus femoris—which are the powerful extensors of the knee joint. Other important stabilizing structures are the *medial* and *lateral collateral ligaments* and the two *cruciate ligaments*. The anterior cruciate originates from the anterior spine of the tibia and attaches to the posterior aspect of the femoral condyle. The *menisci* are the shock absorbers of the knee and are crescentic fibrocartilagenous discs that rest on the periphery of the tibial surface and attach to the joint capsule at their outside edges. Motion at the knee is allowed and restricted by these various ligaments and structures. The anterior knee and posterior popliteal space are best observed with the patient standing, while the rest of the examination of the knee is best performed with the patient supine.

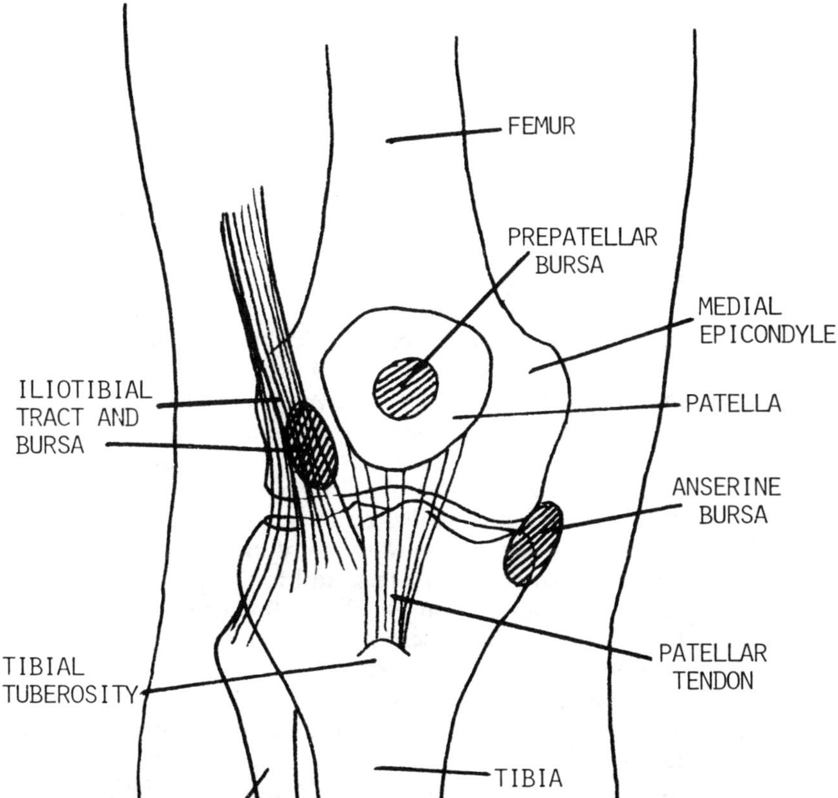

Fig. 18.1. ***Anterior view of right knee.***

II. *Range of Motion at the Knee*
Flexion of 130° and extension at least to 0°. Some patients with genu recurvatum have even greater extension.

Internal and external rotation. After 20° of flexion, gliding and axial rotation are possible so that at 90° of flexion up to 40° of rotation is possible.

III. *Specific regional syndromes*

1. *Joints*

Any of the systemic arthritides may affect the knee, just as any of the infectious agents may infect it. Therefore, as for any other joint, isolated arthritis of the knee must be considered septic until proven otherwise. In children, osteomyelitis of the femur or tibia may resemble acute knee arthritis. Some types of arthritis typically affect the knee to a much greater extent than any other joint. These include hemophilia and pseudogout. *Hemophilic arthritis* is the result of repeated hemarthrosis and injury to the knee and, if untreated, may result in fibrous ankylosis. In these patients, ibuprofen is considered one of the safest non-steroidal anti-inflammatory drugs. Most likely, any of these drugs is safe except aspirin. As for *pseudogout,* knee involvement is as characteristic of it as first MTP arthritis is of gout. Acute onset of knee swelling and pain in the first few days after surgery or after a myocardial infarction is most likely due to pseudogout. Aspiration of the joint to look for the weakly positive birefringent crystals, and for gram stain and culture to exclude infection establishes the diagnosis. *Gout* and the *seronegative spondyloarthropathies* also commonly involve the knee. *Charcot* arthropathy may also involve the knee, most commonly as a complication of tabes dorsalis or diabetes mellitus. The late radiographic appearance of this arthritis is classic.

Baker's cysts formed from extension or herniation of the synovial cavity into the popliteal space are quite common in patients with chronic knee arthritis and effusion for any reason. They can be seen as bulges of the popliteal space with the patient standing. On occasion, they may rupture or dissect distally into the calf. When seen acutely after rupture, the history is usually sufficient to establish the diagnosis. After 24 to 48 hours, the condition may be complicated by secondary development of deep venous thrombosis and phlebitis, in which case treatment for both conditions is needed. For uncomplicated Baker's cyst (even after acute dissection), treatment with a steroid injection into the joint is usually successful. In cases in whom the diagnosis is in question, an ultrasound (if available) or an arthrogram may be needed to establish the diagnosis of an intact or a ruptured Baker's cyst.

Congenital or acquired abnormal alignment of the knees may be seen and may predispose to earlier onset degenerative arthritis. Severe *genu varum* (bow legs) or *genu valgum* (knock knees) may either predispose to or result from degenerative arthritis.

2. *Bursae*

   There are multiple bursae in the area of the knee. The ones most commonly associated with symptoms of bursitis are listed below. *Pes anserine bursitis* involves the bursa at the insertion of the sartorius, gracilis, and semitendinosus tendons into the medial aspect of the proximal tibia. It is often seen in elderly women and may respond to injection with local anesthetic alone. The *prepatellar* bursa when inflamed should be presumed septic. Prolonged kneeling, as seen in housemaids and nuns, is associated with chronic inflammation of this bursa.
3. *Musculotendinous and ligamentous syndromes*
   a. *Patellar tendinitis or jumper's knee* develops from repeated strain to the patellar tendon attachments to the patella. The classic history is worsening patellar pain with jumping, running, or climbing and marked tenderness of the distal poles of the patella.
   b. *Recurrent subluxation and dislocation of the patella* secondary to dynamic or static patellar instability may occur in any age group but is most common in females, especially in their second or third decades. Genu valgum for any reason probably predisposes to it. The patient complains of knee pain, "giving way," swelling, "something slipping out," catching and grinding. Many possible causes have been considered including high-riding patella (or patella alta), abnormalities in alignment, etc. With recurrences, retropatellar crepitation with flexion and extension, and pain on compression of the patella similar to that of chondromalacia patella develops.
   c. Patients with *chondromalacia patella* complain of knee pain with prolonged sitting, climbing stairs, or walk-

ing uphill, and with prolonged walking or running. Irregularities of the posterior surface of the patella are often seen on radiographs.

d. *Iliotibial band contraction/pain*. Vigorous running or hiking may produce pain over the insertion of the iliotibial band. There is point tenderness of this area and the patient limps. Conservative treatment is useful.

e. *Wasting* and *atrophy* of the *quadriceps*, that first involves the vastus medialis and eventually all four extensors, is a common finding in patients with knee pain and worsens the prognosis for preserving function.

f. *Muscle cramps and "charley horses,"* especially in the calf muscles, and at night, are common in pregnant women, elderly patients, following strokes, in association with a number of electrolyte abnormalities and with diuretic use. Quinine sulfate has been used with moderate success, and recently verapamil (a calcium channel blocker) was found to be even more useful.

4. *Neurovascular and compartment syndromes*

Shin splints consist of pain in the anterior foreleg after excessive unaccustomed use. What begins as a dull ache may progress to numbness which extends to the toes. This may also be complicated by muscle sprain of the posterior tibial muscle.

Compartment syndromes may also develop in any of the four compartments of the calf secondary to ischemia of the muscles and impaired arterial and venous flow. If it progresses, worsening pain even at rest with elevation, loss of arterial pulses, and pallor may develop, and surgical decompression becomes necessary.

5. *Bones*

a. *Osteochondritis* of the tibial tubercle (*Osgood-Schlatter's* disease) or of the inferior pole of the patella (*Larsen-Johannson's* disease) may be seen, most commonly in adolescent boys. *Osteochondritis dissecans,* involving small pieces of the articular cartilage that break off in to the joint space, may be seen in males of any age. All of these conditions present with insidious onset of pain. Response to conservative treatment with casting for a few weeks and avoidance of aggravating activities is excellent except for osteochondritis dissecans, which may require surgery.

b. *Fractures* are easily diagnosed with radiographs.

c. *Joint mice.* As a result of osteochondritis dissecans or other injuries, loose bodies (or joint mice) may become free in the synovial cavity with intermittent locking of the knee. It often requires surgery and removal of the fragment(s).

d. *Patello-femoral pain syndrome* is a new term for many of the conditions previously included in the chondromalacia group. Symptoms consist of retropatellar pain that becomes worse with prolonged sitting, going down stairs, or squatting. Treatment is symptomatic and includes strengthening and stretching exercises.

e. *Stress or fatigue* fractures from athletic endeavors may occur, especially in female amenorrheic runners. They can occur anywhere and may not be demonstrable by radiographs taken during the acute episode. In these cases, a bone scan would be diagnostic.

6. *Injuries*

The most common injuries are *strains*. The medial collateral ligament and the medial meniscus are more commonly involved than the lateral structures. "Giving way," whether accompanied by pain or not, usually means ligamentous injury.

Tenderness at the medial or lateral joint space after an injury suggests meniscal or collateral ligament injury as does toe gait with the knee flexed 15°. The McMurray test for a torn meniscus consists of extending the flexed knee while internally or externally rotating the tibia and producing a characteristic click. It is not a reliable test. These and other tests are helpful but not absolutely diagnostic, and arthroscopy or arthrography are usually required for diagnosis when surgical intervention is considered for treatment.

The drawer sign is positive when there is laxity or injury of the cruciate ligaments that allow the tibia to move backward or forward on the femur. Backward laxity suggests posterior cruciate instability, while forward displacement is due to anterior cruciate disruption.

C. EVALUATION

A careful examination of the joints and periarticular structures and, if necessary, weight-bearing AP and lateral radiographs usually suffice.

D. TREATMENT

Avoidance of aggravating factors and use of isometric muscle strengthening exercises are universally helpful. Injection of a topical anesthetic and a steroid preparation is usually helpful as a temporizing measure. Severe degenerative or inflammatory disease, especially in otherwise active individuals over age 50, should be referred for possible surgery.

SUGGESTED READING

1. Cailliet R. *Knee Pain and Disability,* second edition. Philadelphia: F.A. Davis Co., 1983.

Chapter 19

Ankle and Foot Pain

A. REFERRED PAIN

The ankle and foot are not common areas of referred pain, except from a herniated disc, or spinal cord tumor between the L_4-S_3 levels. For all intent and purposes, local injury or inflammation accounts for nearly all cases of ankle and foot pain.

B. REGIONAL AND LOCAL CAUSES OF PAIN

I. *Anatomy and function*

The foot is composed of 26 bones that articulate with the distal surfaces of the tibia and fibula at the ankle. There are multiple joints in the foot which allow us to walk, run, dance ballet, and play soccer. Functionally, the foot is divided into anterior (or forefoot) segment (includes the metatarsals and phalanges); the midfoot (includes the navicular, cuboid, and three cuneiforms), and the posterior segment (includes the talus and calcaneus bones).

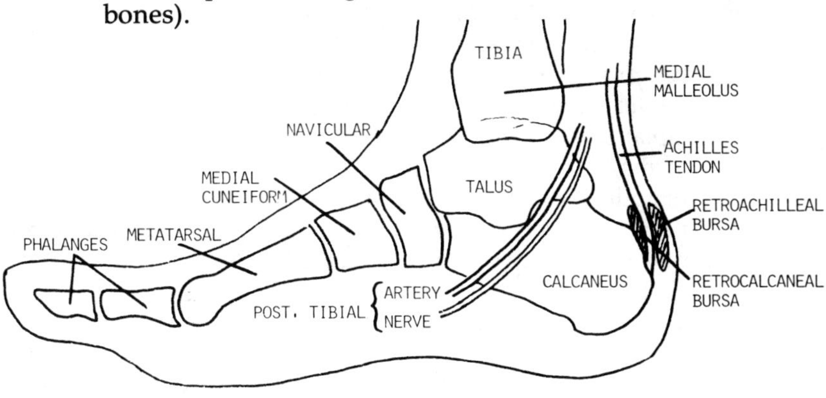

Fig. 19.1. Medial view of foot and ankle.

II. *Range of motion of the ankle and foot include:*

a. *At the ankle* (talocrural joint between the tibia and fibula proximally and the talus distally).
Dorsiflexion 20°, plantar-flexion 50° and same degree of rotation.

b. *Subtalar (or talocalcaneal) joint*
Inversion-elevation of the medial border of the foot as the lateral border depresses 30°, and eversion, the opposite motion, is 20°.

Supination and pronation of the foot combine three subtalar motions: inversion, adduction, and plantar flexion for supination; and eversion, abduction, and dorsiflexion for pronation. The transverse talar joint between the talus and navicular and the calcaneus and cuboid has been termed the surgeon's joint because it is a common site for amputation when forefoot ischemia or infection requires it.

c. *At the MTPs*, flexion and extension facilitates the arch of walking.

Innervation of the foot is from the sciatic nerve via the tibial nerve (medial) and the common peroneal nerve (lateral) and its branch. Several ligaments maintain stability of the ankle and subtalar joints.

III. *Specific Regional Syndromes*

1. *Joints*
The joints in the ankle and foot include the true ankle joint (talocrural) between the distal tibia and fibula and the talus; the subtalar joint, a functional unit that includes the talo-calcaneal joint, and the talo-navicular joint. The midtarsal joints include those between the navicular, cuneiforms, cuboid, and metatarsals. The joints of the forefoot include the metatarsal phalangeal joints and the distal and proximal interphalangeal joints. Almost all of these joints may become involved by an arthritic process, but some are characteristically involved by certain arthritides.

a. *Osteoarthritis* of the first MTP is quite common, especially in older age groups. By age 75, approximately 50% of individuals will have degenerative changes in this joint.

b. *Neuropathic or Charcot joint* is seen in patients with neuropathy and loss of pain and proprioceptive innervation. The foot becomes warm and swollen and, although painful, pain is mild relative to the extensive destruction and disorganization of the joints of the foot, primarily in the midtarsal joints. A "rocker bottom" foot develops with widening of the midfoot. This is most commonly seen in patients with neuropathy secondary to diabetes.

c. *Rheumatoid arthritis* eventually involves all of the synovial lined joints of the foot. Characteristic deformities include pronation and loss of the metatarsal or transverse arch, calcaneus valgus, hallus valgus and fibular deviation of all the toes with pain and calluses under the metatarsal heads. Close to 20% of patients with RA may first present with involvement of the small forefoot joints.

d. *Gout* may involve any joint but characteristically involves the first MTP—"podagra." Tophi are common in the areas near the joints of the feet in patients with tophaceous gout.

e. *Hammer toes*—fixed flexion deformity of the IP joint. Most often affects the second toe. May be congenital or acquired—usually from a pronated foot or from RA. A major concern is finding shoes that provide enough room for the deformed toes.

f. *Hallus rigidus* resulting from osteoarthritis of the first MTP is very painful. The completely fused toe is pain-free, so immobilization of the joint by surgery or a shoe steel bar to keep the MTP from flexing is necessary for treatment.

2. *Bursae*

While there are many bursae in the feet, the three larger and more commonly involved in inflammatory or traumatic bursitis are the *retrocalcaneal* (between the calcaneous insertion and the Achilles tendon), the *superficial bursa* over the Achilles tendon, and the bursa protecting the insertion of the *plantar aponeurosis* or fascia into the inferior distal calcaneus. Any of these bursae may become inflamed. Bursitis of the plantar calcaneal or subcalcaneal bursae may be confused with plantar fascitis. The superficial or retroachilleal bursa is commonly involved secondary to ill-fitting shoes and develops changes known as "pump bumps."

3. *Musculotendinous*
   a. *Dupuytren's contracture* may affect the plantar fascia. As in the hand, it is usually asymptomatic and benign.
   b. *Achilles tendonitis*—the tendon is tender to palpation. Pain is worse with forceful dorsiflexion of the ankle. Pain is similar to that seen with retrocalcaneal bursitis. Either is treated with a short leg walking cast for 3-4 weeks to rest the ankle. Steroid injection may be attempted for bursitis but not for tendonitis because of the risk of tendon rupture.
   c. *Plantar fascitis* is common in runners. Patients present with pain and tenderness at the anteromedial aspect of the calcaneus. The presence of spurs on radiographs *does not* correlate with the clinical syndrome. Plantar fascitis may occur from repetitive trauma, Reiter's syndrome, and psoriatic arthritis, among others.
4. *Neurovascular and entrapment syndromes*
   a. *Sudeck's atrophy or reflex neurodystrophy* of the foot and ankle presents with pain at rest that becomes worse with weight-bearing. The foot is cyanotic or mottled, edematous, cool, tender, moist, and shiny. It usually follows trauma, stroke, or surgery of the hip or knee. It is similar to the syndrome of transient osteoporosis or osteolysis except that in reflex neurodystrophy there are skin changes which are not present in transient osteoporosis.
   b. *Morton's neuroma* is a common interdigital neuritis due to thickening and swelling of a digital nerve. It most commonly occurs between the second and third metatarsal and is most common in middle-aged women. Injection with an anesthetic-steroid mixture usually provides relief, provided there is a change to wider shoes.
   c. *Ischemia of the foot*, whether due to large vessel occlusion from atherosclerosis, vasculitis, small vessel disease from diabetes, or sickle cell disease, is often complicated by leg and foot ulcers that can progress to osteomyelitis

and dry or wet gangrene. Proper footwear and careful hygiene is a very important component of the proper care of these patients.

d. *Common peroneal nerve* injury can occur as the nerve curves around the fibular neck producing weak dorsiflexors and paresthesias of the lateral leg and dorsal foot. If severe enough, it will produce foot drop.

e. *"Tarsal tunnel syndrome,"* secondary to pressure on the posterior tibial nerve as it passes behind and under the medial malleolus, presents with paresthesias in the heel and/or medial or lateral foot depending on the site of entrapment before or after the nerve divides into the medial and lateral plantar nerves.

5. *Bones*

   March fracture is a common stress fracture of a metatarsal following prolonged walking. The foot is tender and slightly swollen on the dorsum, and radiographs initially fail to show the fracture, but as the healing callus forms, it becomes obvious in repeat films. Resting the foot with a walking cast for 3-4 weeks is usually sufficient therapy.

6. *Miscellaneous*

   a. *Pronation of the foot* causes splaying of the metatarsal arch and predisposes to chronic foot strain and pain. Treatment consists of improving the mechanics of the foot by use of a heel wedge on the medial aspect to place the calcaneus in a near vertical position, the Thomas heel. It inverts the heel and supinates the foot. Patients with pronated foot or calcaneal valgus usually give a history of ankle sprains or "weak" ankles. The heel wedge helps to stabilize the pronated foot.

   b. *Metatarsalgia* is pain and tenderness of the plantar heads of the metatarsals. It is usually accompanied by a depressed metatarsal arch with subsequent excess weight-bearing on the 2nd, 3rd, and 4th metatarsal heads. If long-standing, the patient will have thick calluses under the metatarsal heads. Improving the metatarsal transverse arch with an insert, a change to low-heeled shoes, and a metatarsal pad placed proximal to the metatarsal heads are all useful.

c. *Plantaris tendon rupture* produces sudden onset of pain in the heel area. The tendon inserts laterally into the calcaneus or Achilles and extends from the lateral femoral condyle, between the gastrocnemius and soleus muscles. The more common site of rupture is in the midcalf, and may occur during sudden change in step rotation while walking.

d. *Achilles tendon rupture* presents following ankle injury with severe pain in this area and inability to walk. The tear usually occurs within 2″ of the tendon insertion on the calcaneus.

e. *Ankle sprains* are the most common injury and can produce a lot of pain. Treatment is aimed at decreasing swelling. Elevation, ice, and compression bandages are used initially until further evaluation takes place. The deltoid ligament, which stabilizes the medial side of the ankle joint between the tibia, the calcaneus, the fibula and the navicular bones is so strong that in patients with eversion injuries, it avulses the medial malleolus rather than sustain a tear.

C. EVALUATION

While radiographs of the foot and ankle are useful in evaluating joint and bone abnormalities like arthritis or fractures, the history and physical examination are the most important components of the evaluation. Observing the feet at rest and during walking with and without shoes allows us to diagnose the pronated foot, and stressed arches. Checking the foot carefully for areas of callus formation, tenderness, numbness, pulses, and range of motion provides evidence for the specific syndrome.

D. TREATMENT

If the condition is part of a systemic syndrome, systemic treatment is indicated; however, ill-fitting shoes and abnormal gait are quite often involved as well, and this requires improved footwear. For patients with metatarsalgia or calluses over the MTP heads, alteration of the shoes so that the weight on walking can be better distributed is achieved by placement of metatarsal bars proximal to the MTPs. Heel pain from calcaneal bursitis or plantar fasciitis is helped by the use of a soft heel cup. Steroid injection at the inferior calcaneal spur may be done with variable results, depending on the technique of injection and the skill of the physician. For hammer toes and hallus valgus, shoes that are sufficiently wide and deep provide relief. *Surgery should be delayed until other measures fail.*

SUGGESTED READING

1. Cailliet R. *Foot and Ankle Pain,* second edition. Philadelphia: F.A. Davis Co., 1983.

Chapter 20

Sports-Related Injuries in Rheumatology

Seventy percent of millions of recreational athletes and an even higher percentage of competitive or professional athletes will develop a sports-related injury that is severe enough to require intervention. The common forms of sports injury are:

sprain—torn fibers in ligaments
strain—torn fibers in muscle-tendon units
contusion—hemorrhage into muscles
cartilage tear
bone fracture and periostitis

The vast majority of these injuries are caused by inadequate training, faulty technique, biomechanical abnormalities, or overuse and will require no surgical intervention. Recognizing the site and cause of injury and providing conservative medical management of acute and chronic sports-induced problems are roles being filled more and more by rheumatologists.

A. DIAGNOSIS

Many new sports medicine clinics are equipped with videotaping equipment and pressure sensitive treadmills, but a good history and physical examination along with occasional radiographs are adequate tools to make most diagnoses.

History

- —When did symptoms first appear? What exact skeletal movement was being performed?
- —Which activities increase or decrease pain?

—How long has the patient been doing the offending activity and at what level of intensity?
—Recent change in routine or technique?
—Adequate stretching or warm up?
—Types of shoes or other equipment used?
—Has any therapy been effective?

Physical Examination

Extensively examine the injured joint, its neighboring joints, and the contralateral joints for passive, active, and active resisted (against force) ranges of motion. A thorough neurologic examination is also essential. Specific physical examination techniques are described in Chapters 3 and 10 through 19.

Radiographs and Other Tests

Plain films of involved areas may uncover pre-existing musculoskeletal conditions, malalignments, or fractures. Bone scans may show subtle stress fractures or chronic periostitis. Arthroscopy and arthrography may be helpful in recalcitrant cases, who should be referred for orthopedic consultation.

B. TREATMENT

1. *Basic Therapy for Acute Sports Injury*

The majority of strains, sprains, and contusions will respond well to conservative RICE Therapy.

Rest—*No* physical activity or weight-bearing for the injured extremity.

*I*ce and Immobilization—Ice packs are applied to the injury for 30 minutes every three hours while the patient is awake.

Compression—An elastic wrap reduces edema and hematoma formation.

*E*levation—Reduces swelling and pain.

2. *Reconditioning Program for Sports Injury*

After the joint or limb has become asymptomatic, early conservative reconditioning is important to minimize muscle atrophy and joint instability.

—Five minutes of moist heat (shower or towels) to injured area.
—Stretching exercise for 5-10 minutes.
—Alternate hard and gentle exercise for short periods.

—Ice on the previously injured area for 10 minutes after exercise (even if asymptomatic).
—Before bedtime, use heat and stretching exercises for 20 minutes.

SUGGESTED READINGS

1. Brody DM. *Running Injuries: Prevention and management*. Rheumatol Rounds, Summit, New Jersey: Pharmaceuticals Division, CIBA-GEIGY Corp., 1987.

2. Birrer RB. Sports medicine rheumatology. Clin Rheumatol Prac. 1984, 2:196.

3. Neer CS, Loelsch RP. The shoulder in sports. Orthop Clin North Am. 1977, 8:583.

PART III.

SPECIFIC RHEUMATIC SYNDROMES AND DISEASES

Chapter 21

Infectious Arthritis

Almost any pathogen may affect articular and periarticular tissues. A multitude of viruses, bacteria, mycobacteria, mycoplasma, fungi, protozoa, and helminths have been associated with arthritis.

MECHANISMS BY WHICH INFECTIOUS AGENTS PRODUCE ARTHRITIS

1. *Direct joint invasion by the microbe*: The pathogen may invade the joint directly and produce on-going inflammation and destruction. A classic example of this are most of the bacterial pyarthroses. A more recent example is that of Lyme arthritis.
2. *Joints may be affected indirectly as a result of*:
   a. The resulting immune response of the afflicted host. For example, in hepatitis B, circulating immune complexes appear to mediate the polyarthritis that accompanies the prodromal stage of this infection.
   b. Molecular mimicry between the pathogen's antigenic epitopes and similar antigens present in human tissue. The classic example is rheumatic fever secondary to group A beta hemolytic streptococcus and its manifestations of arthritis, carditis, and chorea.
   c. Microbial debris may persist in the joint and perpetuate an inflammatory response, even after the organism is no longer viable in the joint. This is clearly the case in some cases of gonococcal arthritis in which ongoing synovitis is associated with sterile fluid that is inflammatory, so called "post-infectious sterile arthritis." The arthritis slowly resolves over time.
   d. Unknown—This applies to almost all of the reactive arthritides, such as those associated with gastrointestinal infection with

some of the enteric gram-negative organisms (*Shigella, Salmonella, Yersinia,* etc.)

APPROACH TO THE PATIENT WITH SUSPECTED INFECTIOUS ARTHRITIS

Whenever one sees a patient with a suspected infectious arthritis, the following questions should be addressed during the evaluation and therapy of the patient.

1. *What is infected?* The joint, the bursa, the tendons, the bone, or a combination of all four. This will help determine how long to treat. In fact, it is sometimes difficult to make this determination. If you suspect an infectious arthritis but are uncertain if there is only cellulitis, ask for help if available. However, the principle to follow is to tap when in doubt. Even if you are wrong, any organism possibly introduced into the joint from surrounding cellulitis should be rapidly eliminated after antibiotic therapy is begun.
2. *What is the most likely micro-organism involved?* Bacterial infections are much more readily treatable than viral or fungal infections. They are also likely to produce worse damage if not diagnosed early. Culture of the joint, blood cultures, and, when indicated, a cervical or urethral culture for gonococcus should be done. In the patient with a chronic monoarticular arthritis, suspicion of possible TB or fungal infection may require a synovial biopsy and culture for definitive diagnosis. The likely organism will also depend on the characteristics of the population involved, i.e., sexually active, immunocompromised, etc. Finally, the geographic setting will also help narrow the differential of which organism is involved. For example, in Africa, arthritis is a well known frequent presentation of filariasis associated with nocturnal fever, and filariasis is a highly prevalent illness, so in African patients, "parasitic rheumatism" is a likely diagnosis. In the U.S., however, a bacterial or viral etiology would be infinitely more likely.
3. *Does the affected joint contain any foreign objects?* For example, hardware or polymethylmethacrylate cement from joint replacement, thorns, etc. An infected prosthetic joint is always more difficult to manage and cannot be successfully treated if the foreign material is not extensively debrided or removed.
4. *Does the patient belong to a high-risk group?* Patients with long-standing rheumatoid arthritis, patients on chronic steroid therapy, any pa-

tient on immunosuppressive agents, splenectomized patients (including patients with sickle cell anemia), diabetics with foot ulcers, alcoholics, and drug abusers, among others, are at greater risk of infectious arthritis. Each of these groups has a spectrum of microbial susceptibility and a distribution of joint involvement fairly characteristic. For example, while staphylococcus is the most common pathogen overall, in many of these high risk groups gram-negative organisms are also quite common. Therefore, in these groups, early anti-microbial therapy should include agents effective against these organisms until the specific organism is known.

5. *Any other manifestations of infection?* Except in the postoperative patient with a recent joint replacement, most pyarthroses are due to hematogenous spread of the organism from another site such as the urinary tract or the skin. Look for these other sources.
6. *What is the most appropriate therapy?* Does the patient have any allergies, renal or hepatic insufficiency, or any other findings that would require a modification in therapy? Will daily closed drainage of the joint effusion be sufficient or is open drainage necessary? In most cases of bacterial arthritis, intravenous antibiotic and daily closed drainage of the joint to remove bacterial debris and proteolytic enzymes will be sufficient. Open drainage is associated with a worse functional outcome for the joint, but this may in part be related to the more severely affected joints being more likely to require open drainage. Open drainage is necessary in certain joints like the hip.

SUGGESTED READINGS

1. Bennett JC. The infectious etiology of rheumatoid arthritis—new considerations. Arthritis Rheum. 1978; 21:531-8.

2. Bacon PA, Tunn EJ. Infection and arthritis. Quart J. Med. 1986; 61:897-99.

3. Brewerton DA. Causes of arthritis. Lancet. 1988; 2:1063-66.

Chapter 22

Bacterial Infections of the Joints and Periarticular Tissues

Bacteremia is a common occurrence that only infrequently produces consequences. In some patients, bacteremia can lead to septic arthritis. Bacterial arthritis should be considered in any patient who presents with an acutely swollen, hot, and painful joint. It should also be thought of if a similar presentation involves two or more joints, since bacterial arthritis may be oligoarticular, and a delay in diagnosis can be associated with a 25% morbidity and even mortality. This is especially true in patients with underlying rheumatoid arthritis who develop oligoarticular septic arthritis in whom the mortality rate may exceed 50%. While aspiration of the joint is likely to show a high white cell count with a predominance of polymorphonuclear leukocytes, an infected joint may present with few inflammatory changes in the fluid.

BACTERIOLOGIC SPECTRUM OF PYARTHROSES

The bacteriologic spectrum of septic arthritis varies depending on the age and health of the patient. While *Neisseria gonorrhoeae* is the most common organism in the young, sexually active population, *Staphylococcus aureus* is the most common organism in all other settings. In the elderly and debilitated and in those with prosthetic joints, gram negative organisms are also commonly involved. In newborns, *Hemophilus influenzae* is the most likely culprit. Some organisms are well-known for producing an indolent arthritis with few systemic findings of sepsis. *Mycobacterium tuberculosis* is the prototype for this type of arthritis.

However, even *S. aureus* and other pyogens may present without fever and leukocytosis in over half of patients with septic arthritis.

The spectrum of joint involvement also differs among different groups of patients. Overall, the most commonly affected joint is the knee. However, involvement of the sternoclavicular and sacroiliac joints in drug abusers, and of any of the other joints should keep you alert to the possibility that *any* joint can be involved.

In addition to peculiarities of the organism, host factors are also important. Prosthetic joints, alcoholism, intravenous drug use, old age, underlying rheumatoid arthritis or other chronic illness, and some therapies (like steroids) predispose and modify the response to the infecting organism.

SPECIFIC PYARTHROSES SYNDROMES

1. *Gonococcal arthritis*

   The gonococcus is particularly likely to infect a joint during bacteremia, even in otherwise healthy adults without any other predisposing factor. The arthritis may be a migratory polyarthritis that presents with fever and dermatitis (about 60%), or a purulent arthritis (30-40%) similar to that seen in non-gonococcal bacterial arthritis. The joint fluid may be sterile, and the gonococcemia may be missed, so in any sexually active patient with purulent arthritis, or tenosynovitis and splinter-like lesions in the extremities, culture of the cervix, oropharynx, and/or urethra for gonococcus should be done in addition to culture of the joint fluid and blood. A similar presentation may occur with meningococcus, although this is quite uncommon except in patients with deficiencies of some complement proteins in serum.

   Gonococcal arthritis may evolve into a post-infectious phase during which the effusion is sterile, but there is ongoing inflammation due to remaining bacterial cell products, most likely peptidoglycans from the bacterial cell wall. It improves slowly despite antibiotic therapy and daily aspiration of reaccumulated joint fluid. Unlike arthritis with non-gonococcal organisms, joint destruction is quite rare in patients with gonococcal arthritis, even in those whose joints are culture-positive.
2. *Prosthetic joint infections*

   These can be classified according to the time after surgery when they occur. (a) *Early* or *acute* infections are those that occur within

12 weeks of surgery and account for 40% of total infections. They are usually due to contamination of the joint and/or prosthesis or cement (methylmethacrylate) with the organism at the time of surgery, most commonly *S. aureus* or *S. epidermidis*. (b) *Subacute* infection occurs within a year of implantation but later than 12 weeks and 45% of total infections fall into this category. (c) *Late* infections occur one year or longer after surgery and are almost always due to hematogenous spread of an organism and subsequent seeding of the prosthetic joint. They comprise 15% of the cases. In late infections, the organism may be any of those found in urinary tract infections, bronchitis, pneumonia, etc.

The incidence of early infections may be reduced by using perioperative antibiotic prophylaxis with an anti-staphylococcal drug 20 minutes before surgery and for 24 hours thereafter. Likewise, the use of filtered laminar air flow in the operating room, especially when accompanied by whole-body exhaust ventilated suits for the operating team, further reduces the risk of infection. Any infectious processes, even if asymptomatic, must be successfully treated preoperatively in patients scheduled for prosthetic surgery. Antibiotic-impregnated cement has also been tried to prevent a septic prosthetic joint. Gentamicin is the antibiotic most frequently used because it is least likely to sensitize the patient and yet has activity against the most likely organisms.

Patients with prosthetic joints who are at greatest risk of infection are those of advanced age, in poor health, with previous surgery at the site of the prosthesis, and who were previously treated with corticosteroids.

3. *Intravenous Drug Abusers*

In heroin users, fibro-cartilagenous joints are preferentially involved and may present with only pain in the joint without any systemic symptoms of infection like fever and leukocytosis. Sacroiliac, sternocostal, sternoclavicular, pubic symphysis, and the knee joints are the joints most commonly involved. Although *S. aureus* accounts for three-quarters of the cases, fungal arthritis with *Candida* species, and pseudomonas arthritis are also seen in this group. Because of the types of joints often involved, joint aspiration may be unsuccessful in these patients, and open biopsy may be required for diagnosis.

BACTERIAL BURSITIS

This nearly always affects the superficial bursae, especially the prepatellar and olecranon bursae. Infection is commonly due to local trauma, and the organisms responsible are *Staphylococcus aureus* (80%) or group A streptococcus (10%). The populations at greatest risk are those in certain occupations in which there is repetitive trauma to the bursae like carpet-laying, roofing, plumbing, gardening, and some sports including gymnastics and playing football on artificial turf. Patients with chronic lung disease and those on chronic dialysis who exert frequent pressure on their elbow are also prone to traumatize it with subsequent bacterial bursitis—"lunger's elbow" and "dialysis elbow."

Diagnosis is established by aspiration, white count, Gram stain, and culture of the infected bursae. These patients may maintain a fairly good range of motion of the joint as opposed to those with a septic joint. Physical examination is useful in determining whether the bursa or the joint is involved. Treatment with antibiotics may be either oral or parenteral, depending on the degree of illness and debility. Bactericidal antibiotics with good coverage for staphylococcus are preferred and are given for 7-14 days. Surgical removal of the infected bursa is rarely indicated.

APPROACH TO THE PATIENT WITH A SUSPECTED SEPTIC JOINT OR BURSA

1. Consider it in any patient presenting with an acute or subacute arthritis and in patients with a chronic monoarthritis.
2. Aspirate the synovial fluid from affected joints for cell count and differential, Gram stain and culture, and to look for crystals. If the setting is suggestive, culture for fungi and mycobacteria, or do extra-articular cultures for gonococcus. The gram stain is very helpful when positive but is often non-diagnostic, so a clinical "best guess" is made.
3. Blood cultures are indicated in any acutely ill patient. They may demonstrate the pathogen even when joint fluid is sterile.
4. For initial coverage, choose one or more antibiotics that are active against the most likely *and* most dangerous pyogens. This means choosing a drug with activity against *S. aureus,* and *N. gonorrhoeae.* In patients with prosthetic or traumatized joints and in intravenous

drug users, gram-negative coverage (including *Pseudomonas*) is also indicated until the organism responsible is identified. In teenagers (and rarely in adults), *H. influenzae* can be the culprit. Intra-articular antibiotics are generally of no value.

5. Frequent closed aspirations of the joint to decrease the volume of pus and organisms is helpful and should be done daily so long as an effusion is present. Following serial white counts and culture of the fluid help to determine efficacy of therapy. If after 7-10 days the joint aspiration is still culture positive, open drainage should be considered. For hip joints, open drainage may be best. The prognosis for joint recovery is lowest for the hip, and best for gonococcal arthritis. Bedrest should only be prescribed as needed, but splinting and rest periods are helpful during the acute inflammation.
6. Physical therapy to maintain as much of the normal range of motion of the joint as possible should be started as soon as the acute inflammation subsides in 5-7 days.
7. Prophylactic anticoagulation if the patient is not ambulatory should be instituted to prevent the development of deep venous thrombosis and pulmonary embolism.

RECOMMENDATIONS FOR ANTIMICROBIAL THERAPY IN SEPTIC ARTHRITIS OR BURSITIS IN ADULTS
(The safety of the recommended agents in pregnant patients should be confirmed with the obstetrician.)

Most antibiotics achieve excellent concentration in the joint fluid. Aminoglycosides lose activity with increasing acidity in the fluid; consequently, in effusions with a high concentration of polymorphonuclear leukocytes and associated low pH, aminoglycosides will achieve less efficient concentrations. Our recommendations in non-allergic patients with normal renal function are as follows (doses would have to be modified in patients with renal insufficiency), but other antibiotic regimens may be equally effective.

a. In a sexually active patient without factors predisposing to gram negative bacillary arthritis, *ceftriaxone 2 gm IV or IM every 24 hours.* Other more narrow spectrum and/or less expensive antibiotics may be substituted after the organism is identified and its antibiotic susceptibility determined.

b. In a similar patient not requiring hospital admission: *ampicillin* 3.5 gm p.o. OR *amoxicillin* 3 gm p.o. *PLUS probenecid 1 gm p.o.* followed by *500 mg p.o. q.i.d.* of amoxicillin or ampicillin for seven days or more.
c. In a patient at high risk of infection with a methicillin-resistant staphylococcus (e.g., drug abusers in some communities and nosocomial infectious arthritis) or with *Pseudomonas*, use *ceftazidime 2 gm IV q. 8 hours,* and *vancomycin 1 gm IV q. 12 hours for 48 hours.* As mentioned earlier, narrower spectrum, less expensive antibiotics should be substituted as soon as the causative organism(s) is(are) identified.

   Treatment varies from 7-14 days for gonococcal arthritis to six months to a year for tuberculous arthritis. Most non-gonococcal bacterial arthritis should be treated for 4-6 weeks or until the inflammation has disappeared.

OSTEOMYELITIS

Infection of a bone may occur in any part of the skeletal system in any patient at any time. The bacteriologic spectrum is similar to that of the bacterial pyarthroses with *S. aureus* accounting for the great majority of cases. In children, it commonly presents as joint pain in the knee. The pathogenesis is either bacteremia with localization to bone, or direct penetration of bone secondary to trauma, such as open fractures, contiguous infection as in diabetic foot ulcers, or breakdown of skin as seen in pressure sores. The presentation may be acute or chronic. In general, the healthier the patient the more likely it is that he or she will present acutely.

Diabetic patients with osteomyelitis from a foot ulcer usually have a more subacute or chronic history and polymicrobial infection with gram positive cocci, gram negative rods, and anaerobes. In *drug addicts*, subacute or chronic osteomyelitis due to a *Pseudomonas* species is a well-recognized syndrome. *Tubercular* osteomyelitis most commonly involves the vertebral bodies (Pott's disease), develops slowly (over months to over a year), and is usually associated with a paravertebral mass from an abscess. Treatment with two or more antituberculous drugs for up to two years is recommended after establishing the diagnosis with tissue culture. *Sickle cell anemia* patients are particularly susceptible to joint and bone infection with non-typhoidal *Salmonella*, so while the cultures are pending, coverage should include an antibiotic with activity against these organisms.

Except for soft-tissue swelling, the plain radiographs in acute osteomyelitis may be normal during the first 7-14 days. If the suspicion is high, a technetium bone scan (which lights up areas of increased vascularity) or a gallium scan (which concentrates in areas with high concentration of polymorphonuclear leukocytes) can be helpful. By two weeks or more, typical changes of irregular lytic areas and periosteal elevation can be detected on plain films. By four weeks, typical reactive sclerosis becomes obvious.

Treatment can be difficult when the condition is long-standing because of the tendency for osteomyelitis to produce isolated nonvascularized areas of bone (called sequestrae) that may contain many organisms but not be reachable by the antibiotics present in serum. In addition, the tendency of osteomyelitis to be chronic or to appear cured only to relapse several years later is well known. Treatment of the commonly found organisms like *S. aureus* and the gram negative rods is usually given for six weeks until the bone appears healed by radiographs or the patient is asymptomatic and any drainage previously present disappears. The sedimentation rate may take up to three or more months to return to normal, and some authorities recommend extending the treatment period accordingly.

The recent advent of the quinolones (ciprofloxacin and others) with their ability to reach excellent concentrations in bone when given orally have provided relief from prolonged parenteral treatment of aerobic gram-positive and -negative organisms. Unfortunately, these drugs have poor activity against anaerobic species. Doses of 750 mg p.o. b.i.d. of ciprofloxacin have been effective. Lower dosages are sufficient in patients with renal insufficiency. In diabetics with foot osteomyelitis, where anaerobes play an important role, ciprofloxacin can be used in combination with doses of metronidazole of 500-750 mg p.o. t.i.d. quite successfully.

At the time of this writing, a couple of case reports have appeared suggesting that ciprofloxacin may be capable of inducing an acute inflammatory arthritis. This association needs to be confirmed more broadly, but meanwhile, keep this consideration in mind as one of many possible causes of arthritis in a patient with osteomyelitis taking this agent. In addition, this drug may adversely affect theophylline metabolism and anti-convulsant effects. Beware of these potential problems.

SUGGESTED READINGS

1. Goldenberg DL, Reed JI. Bacterial arthritis. N Engl J Med. 1985; 312:764-71.

2. Ho G Jr, Mikolich DJ. Bacterial infection of the superficial subcutaneous bursae. Clin Rheum Dis. 1986; 12:437-57.

3. Brause BD. Infections associated with prosthetic joints. Clin Rheum Dis. 1986; 523-36.

4. Editorial. Bacterial arthritis. Lancet. 1986; 2:721-2.

Chapter 23

Arthritis Associated with Viral Infections

Multiple viruses have been implicated in the development of arthritis, and even more commonly, arthralgias, either through direct tissue tropism for synovium (e.g., rubella), or through more indirect mechanisms like immune complex arthritis (e.g., hepatitis B).

Most viral arthritides are self-limited and of short duration. Indeed, the ARA criteria for rheumatoid arthritis (RA) requires that the articular symptoms be present for at least six weeks before entertaining the diagnosis of RA, since presumably, most self limited viral associated articular symptoms resolve within six weeks. In actual fact, some patients with viral associated arthritis may continue to have articular symptoms for months or even years, depending on the specific virus and the individual patient. To date, however, none of these patients have been found to go on to develop an erosive destructive arthritis of the type seen with far-advanced RA.

VIRAL INFECTIONS ASSOCIATED WITH ARTHRITIS

These include some single-stranded RNA viruses like rubella and the alpha viruses, some DNA viruses, and a retrovirus.

1. *Rubella*
   Rubella is a small single-stranded RNA virus. Both the wild virus strains and the strains used in the vaccine can produce arthritis which is usually limited to adult women without prior exposure. The incidence of joint manifestations in children is very low compared to up to 3% of females and 6% of males during rubella epidemics. The vaccine has been associated with arthritis in up to 5%

of children and in more adult women than men. With the newer vaccine, arthritis has been found in close to 15% of vaccinated women. The incidence of arthropathy was higher with the earlier vaccines.

The presentation commonly includes carpal tunnel syndrome and the arthritis involves the small joints of the hands and feet in a symmetrical distribution. Short-lasting low grade fever, rash, and lymphadenopathy usually accompany the arthritis. The arthritis seen following infection with the wild strain is self-limited and resolves within a few weeks. In contrast, recurrence and greater severity of joint symptoms is more common following vaccine-associated arthritis. Diagnosis is based on the history of recent vaccination or exposure and can be confirmed serologically. Treatment is symptomatic.

2. *Human Parvovirus B19*

This virus has now been established as the cause for "fifth disease" or erythema infectiosum ("slapped cheek syndrome") in children. It is a very small single-stranded DNA virus which appears to be ubiquitous in many populations. It was found by chance while evaluating new tests for hepatitis B surface antigen. During the next 10 years, its role as the cause for aplastic crises in patients with hemoglobinopathies was discovered, and later it was established as the etiologic agent in fifth disease. Over 50% of adults in most populations studied have antibodies to it. Infection usually occurs before age 10.

When infection first occurs in adulthood, small joint polyarthralgias and arthritis sometimes in association with a short-lived rash are the presenting symptoms. The arthritis is usually self-limited but may be prolonged as long as five years. Most infections are epidemic, but sporadic cases are also common. A related human *Parvovirus*, "RA-1," was isolated from the synovium of a patient with classic seropositive RA. How significant this agent may be in other RA patients remains to be established. Treatment, as for most viral infections, is symptomatic.

3. *Hepatitis B arthritis*

This virus was one of the first reported associations between a viral infection and a rheumatic disease. A small joint symmetrical polyarthritis, additive or migratory, predominantly affecting women, can develop prior to the onset of jaundice in 10-25% of patients. The illness is self-limited (1-3 weeks) and may be accompanied by a rash. During the time of joint symptoms, hepatitis B surface antigen circulates in excess, and circulating immune complexes are thought to be pathogenic in this syndrome. Other rheumatic associations with hepatitis B infection include a subset of polyarteritis nodosa and mixed essential cryoglobulinemia. Diagnosis can be made by testing for the antigens and antibodies of hepatitis B in serum, and treatment is symptomatic.

4. *Human immunodeficiency virus* (HIV-1)
This recently identified single-stranded RNA retrovirus of the lenti group is the cause of acquired immunodeficiency syndrome (AIDS) and AIDS-related complex (ARC). Recent reports suggest that it can be associated with musculoskeletal manifestations. A prospective study of 101 patients with AIDS identified 72 among them with musculoskeletal manifestations. These manifestations included enthesopathies like Reiter's syndrome and psoriatic arthritis, as well as arthralgias, myositis, myalgias, and one patient with vasculitis. These patients had no serologic evidence of autoimmunity and the pathogenesis of these manifestations is unclear. None of the musculoskeletal manifestations were specific for AIDS with the possible exception of a very severe migratory oligoarticular pain syndrome sometimes accompanied by arthritis. These symptoms often respond to treatment with zidovudine (AZT).

5. *The alpha virus groups*
Includes all of the viruses known to produce epidemic arthritis. They are single-stranded RNA viruses that have a distinct geographic distribution, although there is evidence of ongoing spread to other parts of the world. The major ones are Chikungunya, Sindbis, and O'nyong-nyong, mostly in Africa and Asia; Ross River virus in Australia and the South Pacific; Mayaro virus in South America: and a Sindbis-related virus in Sweden and Finland.

Most produce polyarthralgias lasting between a few days to 3-4 weeks, some polyarticular and symmetrical, others oligoarticular and asymmetric. The clinical presentation usually consists of rash, fever, and arthritis. There is no treatment for these syndromes except symptomatic therapy.

SUGGESTED READINGS

1. Smith CA, Woolf AD, Lenci M. Parvoviruses: Infections and arthropathies. Clin Rheum Dis. 1987; 13:249-63.

2. Berman A, Espinoza LR, Diaz JD, et al. Rheumatic manifestations of human immunodeficiency virus infection. Am J Med. 1988; 85:59-64.

3. Fraser JRE. Epidemic polyarthritis and Ross River virus disease. Clin Rheum Dis. 1986; 12:369-88.

4. Kaye BR. Rheumatologic manifestations of infection with human immunodeficiency virus (HIV). Ann Intern Med. 1989; 111:158-67.

Chapter 24

Rheumatic Fever

Rheumatic fever is a multisystem clinical syndrome that follows pharyngeal infection with some strains of group A beta-hemolytic streptococci in susceptible individuals. It has variable but predictable clinical manifestations that appear between one week (arthritis) and several months (chorea) after the pharyngitis. Although migratory polyarthritis is one of the most common symptoms, the worse morbidity results from carditis and its late sequelae of rheumatic valvular disease. Until the last few decades, rheumatic heart disease was the leading cause of morbidity and mortality among the young and middle-aged population in this country, and this is still true in the underdeveloped countries of the world.

The incidence of rheumatic fever in the United States dropped dramatically following World War II, to the point that few of the recent medical school graduates have ever seen or diagnosed a case. In the last few years, however, several epidemics of rheumatic fever have been reported from several areas of our country. The clinical manifestations appear similar to the disease seen decades ago, although the Utah epidemic appeared to have a very high incidence of carditis. This may be a reflection of patient referral and selection. The population involved appears to have changed. Instead of affecting the over-populated and crowded poor ethnic minorities of the inner cities, the recent epidemics have affected white, affluent, suburban or rural youngsters. One of the recent epidemics occurred in young adult military recruits, in much the same pattern as was earlier observed in similar populations in the 1940s. Contrary to what was once thought, the clinical characteristics of the disease are the same in any climate and in any country.

PATHOGENESIS

The evidence that rheumatic fever is pathogenetically related to prior throat infection with certain rheumatogenic M type highly mucoid strains of group A beta-hemolytic streptocci comes from several observations.

a. Epidemics of rheumatic fever (RF) were noted to follow epidemics of pharyngitis with certain streptococci. Studies during epidemics showed an incidence of RF of 1-3% in military recruits and other populations following throat infection.
b. Although up to one-third to one-half of patients with either first onset RF or recurrence do not recall a prior sore throat, nearly all patients with rheumatic fever (except some patients with chorea) have serologic evidence of recent infection with group A streptococci.
c. In addition, studies of antibodies to type-specific streptococci showed some cross-reactivity (molecular mimicry) with antigens present in heart and brain tissues.
d. Finally, the strongest supportive evidence came from trials that showed the efficacy of primary and secondary antibiotic prophylaxis in reducing or eliminating the risk of rheumatic fever.

DIAGNOSIS

There is no diagnostic test for rheumatic fever. As early as the 1930s and early 1940s, the constellation of clinical findings in RF was noted and formalized by Dr. T. Duckett Jones, who proposed a set of major and minor criteria to establish the diagnosis. As the epidemiology of rheumatic fever evolved, the criteria were modified in 1955, revised in 1965, and revised again most recently in 1984. They are discussed below. In summary, the diagnosis is made when two major or one major and two minor criteria are present, *if* there is supporting evidence of a preceding group A streptococcal infection *and* if other conditions that may mimic it are ruled out.

I. *Major Criteria*
   1. *Arthritis*. The typical joint involvement is a migratory polyarthritis that involves mostly the middle-sized peripheral joints (knees, ankles, wrists, elbows) but may involve any. A few joints at a time are involved for a few days and resolve completely

while other joints become involved. It is the most frequent manifestation, present in about 75% of patients during the initial attack. Arthritis is also the first manifestation, occurring 1-5 weeks after the pharyngeal infection. Ulnar deviation of the fingers at the MCPs without arthritis (Jaccoud's arthritis) may be seen years later, more commonly in association with rheumatic heart disease than with earlier rheumatic arthritis.

2. *Carditis*. This is a pancarditis. The endocardium, particularly the valvular structures, are the most severely affected. Pericardial effusion is seen but subsequent constrictive pericarditis is not. There is evidence that patients who do not develop valvular damage during the initial attack are not susceptible to ongoing "silent" damage or to valvular involvement during subsequent attacks. The incidence of carditis varies from epidemic to epidemic but is probably near 50%. The major risks from RF are due to carditis, and patients with cardiomegaly and congestive heart failure during the acute attack are at risk of death. Survivors have a 50% risk of developing a recurrence during the five years following the illness, and this risk decreases over the next five years and stabilizes at 10% thereafter. The characteristic histologic finding is the Aschoff nodule.

   Clinically, murmurs of mitral regurgitation and aortic regurgitation predict valvular involvement. A characteristic diastolic low-pitched murmur coincident with a third heart sound and best heard at the apex in full expiration with the patient lying on his left side is the Carey-Coombs murmur. Electrocardiographic changes like prolongation of the PR interval or delayed conduction are often seen but are not specific. Of all four valves, the mitral valve is the one most commonly affected with resulting mitral insufficiency and stenosis. The valve scars in the shape of a "fish mouth," which is quite characteristic. The aortic valve may also be affected, and the tricuspid is only rarely involved. While hemodynamic changes due to valvular stenosis or incompetence are a major long term cause of morbidity and mortality, bacterial endocarditis is a risk anytime there is a focus of infection and bacteremia. In addition, recurrences are associated with worsening valve damage.

3. *Erythema marginatum*. This is a serpiginous evanescent erythematous rash of the trunk and proximal extremities that

may be unnoticed by the patient. Heat can bring it on. Although characteristic, it is not specific. It is an uncommon manifestation that may be present intermittently for months after the acute attack.

4. *Chorea* (also called Sydenham's chorea, chorea minor, and St. Vitus dance) is rare. It never presents in sexually mature males, can affect boys and girls and, rarely, women. It may last from two months to as long as three years and is characterized by very abrupt movements of the extremities and face. Mood disturbances commonly accompany and may precede the chorea. The onset of chorea is usually delayed enough (1-6 months) that conclusive evidence of prior group A strep infection is often lacking by the time the patient comes to medical attention.
5. *Subcutaneous nodules*. These are uncommon except in association with rheumatic heart disease. They tend to occur over bony prominences and extensor tendons and usually last a few days. They are not tender.

II. *Minor Criteria*

These include known prior rheumatic fever or rheumatic heart disease, fever, arthralgias, presence of acute phase reactants in serum (C-reactive protein and elevated ESR) and prolonged PR interval by ECG.

III. *Evidence of prior Group A infection*

1. *Positive throat culture*. This is usually negative by the time the RF appears. Conversely, asymptomatic carriers may develop a few symptoms similar to RF but secondary to some other illness.
2. *Elevated single titer* or *greater than two tube dilution rise* in simultaneously performed serologic tests for streptococcal antibodies. The anti-streptolysin O test is more commonly used. When available, the level of the anti-DNAse B is also useful. However, infection with non-rheumatic streptococci can also elevate the titers, so an elevated level alone is not sufficient for the diagnosis. The magnitude of the antibody response has been associated with the attack rate of RF.

IV. *Differential diagnosis*

This includes any febrile illness that can produce arthritis, including gonococcal bacteremia, bacterial endocarditis, serum sickness and other circulating immune complex diseases, sickle cell disease, and rheumatoid arthritis among others.

PRIMARY AND SECONDARY TREATMENT AND PROPHYLAXIS

Antibiotic therapy similar to that recommended for streptococcal pharyngitis (10-day course of oral penicillin VK 250 mg q.i.d. or, if penicillin allergic, oral erythromycin 250 mg q.i.d.) is given, plus a regimen of once monthly intramuscular benzathine penicillin G 1.2 million units as secondary prophylaxis through at least age 30 to prevent RF recurrence. Oral daily prophylaxis may be preferred in the form of 1 gm sulfadiazine q.d., or 200,000 units of penicillin b.i.d. between meals.

When the incidence of RF was high, follow-up cultures of the patient as well as cultures of contacts and treatment of carriers to prevent colonization and infection with the dreaded streptococcus were recommended. As RF became less common, this practice was discontinued for several years. The 1986-87 report of 10 recruits with RF at a San Diego naval training site, six additional cases of group A streptococcal pneumonia among these recruits, and septic arthritis in yet another one, led to reinstitution of the policy of primary prophylaxis of all recruits with a one time dose of benzathine penicillin G 1.2 million units IM.

Other treatment may include salicylates and steroids as well as specific treatment for heart failure, chorea, etc. However, because of the remarkable and predictable response of the illness to therapeutic levels of salicylates, it is very important that you *withhold* treatment with salicylates until the disease is completely expressed so as to avoid confusion regarding the diagnosis. Low doses of codeine may be used for symptomatic treatment.

SUGGESTED READINGS

1. Ad Hoc Committee to Revise the Jones Criteria (modified) of the Council on Rheumatic Fever and Congenital Heart Disease of the American Heart Association: Jones Criteria (revised) for guidance in the diagnosis of rheumatic fever. Circulation 1984; 69:204A-208A.

2. Bisno AL, Shulman ST, Dajani AS. The rise and fall (and rise?) of rheumatic fever. JAMA 1988; 259:728-9.

3. Feinstein AR. On blind men, elephants, spectrums, and controversies: lessons from rheumatic fever revisited. J Chron Dis. 1986; 39:337-42.

Chapter 25

Lyme Disease

In 1975, two mothers from Old Lyme, Connecticut, each with a child recently diagnosed with juvenile rheumatoid arthritis (JRA) noticed that several other children in their neighborhood had also been diagnosed with JRA. One of the mothers herself, her husband and a second child had also been affected with arthritis. One mother contacted the rheumatology division at Yale University and the other the State Health Department. In less than 10 years, thanks to the rapid and persistent investigative efforts of these two groups, the cause, clinical spectrum, and effective treatment of this disease were elucidated.

EPIDEMIOLOGY

Lyme disease is one of the tick-borne spirochetoses and the most common of all tick-borne illnesses. It is caused by the newly described *Borrelia burgdorferi*, a spirochete that more closely resembles *B. hermsii* (which produces relapsing fever) than species of *Treponema* and *Leptospira* that can also produce disease in humans. Despite the close taxonomy, Lyme spirochete does not lead to the production of antireaginic antibody (i.e., VDRL).

Lyme disease has been reported primarily in this country and Europe but has a world-wide distribution. In the United States, it occurs most frequently from spring through late fall. The spirochete can be transmitted by several of the "hard" ticks and also by some fleas. The disease has been reported from almost every state of the Union, although it clusters around the northeastern states, Wisconsin, and Minnesota. The cases in Connecticut were traced to infected nymphs of the *Ixodes dammini* ticks carried by many of the white-footed mice and white-tailed deer prevalent in the woods and sand dunes of these areas.

CLINICAL SYNDROME AND DIAGNOSIS

The disease is thought to have three stages (although some favor a simpler characterization of "early" and "late" disease).

Stage 1. Occurs within one day to four weeks after the tick bite and is manifested by constitutional flu-like symptoms and fatigue, plus the characteristic rash—erythema chronicum migrans (ECM). Headache, low-grade fever, chills, myalgias, arthralgias, backache, and lymphadenopathy are common during this stage. A small group of patients may present with hepatic pain, anorexia, nausea, and vomiting suggestive of hepatitis.

ECM was once used to identify patients with Lyme disease but as the clinical spectrum of the disease has evolved, it may not be present in 30-40% of patients. ECM starts as a red macule or papule that later looks like a red ring with a usually flat central clearing that may be indurated. These lesions often occur at the site of tick bites and can range in size up to 70 cm or may be multiple and located in sites away from the original bite. The lesion results from peripheral migration of the spirochete which can be demonstrated in histologic sections and cultured from the lesion. Other less specific rashes have also been described including an annular rash uncommonly malar in distribution that spares the palms and soles. A small erythematous vesicular rash with central clearing can also occur.

The clinical evolution varies. Among 55 patients with ECM who were not treated with antibiotics and were followed prospectively for three to eight years (mean of six years), 20% had complete resolution, 18% had intermittent articular, periarticular, or musculoskeletal pain, 51% had intermittent episodes of frank arthritis (some polyarticular), and 11% developed chronic arthritis.

Effective antibiotic treatment of Stage 1 will shorten the duration of the rash and either prevent or ameliorate Stage 2 and 3 disease. However, antibodies to the spirochete do not develop for about two months after the tick bite, so the serology is not helpful during this stage, and, in the absence of the pathognomonic rash, the disease can be difficult to diagnose. The laboratory findings are not diagnostic and likewise only reflect an acute inflammatory response of varying degrees. Liver enzymes may also be increased.

Antibiotic treatment during this stage may abrogate the serologic immune response without completely eliminating the organism. This "sero-negative Lyme disease" is responsive to more effective antibiotic treatment and has been confirmed by specific tests of cellular immunity.

Stage 2. Develops 3 weeks to 5 months after the tick bite. Cardiac, neurological, ophthalmological and musculoskeletal findings may occur. The neurologic triad of lymphocytic meningo-encephalitis, polyradiculitis and cranial nerve palsies (especially Bell's palsy) is characteristic. This triad is not always present, and other neurologic manifestations have been seen, including transverse myelitis, mononeuritis multiplex, and other findings compatible with multiple sclerosis. Ten percent of patients develop cardiac manifestations, primarily heart block at the AV node. Close to one-half of these patients require temporary pacemakers. Uveitis is very rare but has been reported.

Diagnosis at this stage and in Stage 3 can be established by the presence of antibodies to the Lyme spirochete by immunofluorescence or ELISA. Unfortunately, in endemic areas, anywhere from a few to near 25% of asymptomatic individuals may have positive serology for Lyme spirochete due to previous exposure. The method used for detecting the antibody may be responsible for these findings, with some assays being less specific for active infection than others.

Stage 3. Occurs five months to years after the tick bite. The skin, the joints, and the nervous system may be affected. The *arthritis* is usually monoarticular or oligoarticular, or may be a migratory polyarthritis lasting a few months with resolution and later recurrence. The knee and other mid-sized joints (including the temporomandibular joint) are most often affected, but any joint may be involved, including the small joints of the hands or feet. A small percentage of these patients go on to develop a chronic arthritis, usually involving one or both knees with pannus formation and rheumatoid arthritis-like histology. An arteritis with onion-skinning of vessels appears to be a specific finding.

In about one-quarter of patients in Stage 3, spirochetes can be identified in the tissue by Dieterle silver stain. Patients who are HLA-DR4 and/or DR2 may be at increased risk of developing the arthritis. The pathogenesis appears to be directly related to ongoing presence of viable spirochetes in the joint.

The *neurologic* findings are suggestive of multiple sclerosis, and a recent case of focal encephalitis in a young woman six years after Lyme disease suggests the possibility of delayed recurrence of other neurologic deficits. The *skin* changes included a long-recognized dermatitis seen in Europe—acrodermatitis chronica atrophicans, which in the late stages resembles morphea. Isolated morphea has also been reported in association with late stage Lyme disease.

DIAGNOSIS

As reviewed above, the diagnosis can be difficult in some patients. The Center for Disease Control suggests the following criteria:

Endemic area: ECM or antibody titer of 1:256 or above and involvement of one or more of the following organ systems: musculoskeletal, neurological, or cardiac.

Non-endemic area: ECM with antibody titer equal to or above 1:256, *or* ECM with involvement of two or more of the organ systems above, *or* an antibody titer equal to or above 1:256 and manifestations in one or more organ system.

As mentioned earlier, some patients treated with antibiotics during Stage 1 (ECM stage) may never mount an antibody response and may develop Stage 3 disease that responds to a longer course of antibiotics. In these patients, there is evidence of cell-mediated immunity to the Lyme spirochete. Reports of similar response in presumably negative controls may represent earlier unknown exposure or test inaccuracy. Better standardization from lab to lab of serologic tests are ongoing.

TREATMENT

Early disease in adults is treated with tetracycline 250 mg p.o. q.i.d. for 10-12 days, or phenoxymethylpenicillin 500 mg p.o. q.i.d. for 14-21 days. For the late stages, penicillin G sodium 3.3 million units intravenously q. 4 hours for 10 days has been shown to work, and so has doxycycline 100 mg b.i.d. for 30 days. In patients who do not respond, ceftriaxone 2 gm intravenously twice a day for 14 days has been effective.

RECOMMENDATIONS

The places most likely to harbor infected ticks are areas of vegetation like dunes, tall grass, woods, and brush. Visitors should avoid them and, when visiting endemic areas, wear clothing that does not allow ticks to go between it and the skin. Check the body, especially dark areas such as skin folds, for ticks and remove any straight up with tweezers. Transmission of the spirochete while the tick feeds on the human host takes close to 24 hours, so twice daily checking for ticks should provide sufficient time to avoid infection.

SUGGESTED READINGS

1. Steere AC, Schoen RT, Taylor E. The clinical evolution of Lyme arthritis. Ann Intern Med. 1987; 107:725-31.

2. Goldings EA, Gericho J. Lyme Disease. Rheum Dis Clin NA. 1986; 12:343-67.

3. Steere AC. Lyme disease. N Engl J Med. 1989; 321:586-96

Chapter 26

Rheumatoid Arthritis

Rheumatoid arthritis (RA) is a systemic disease characterized by a predominantly symmetrical inflammatory polyarthritis. It is the most common of the inflammatory arthritides, affecting about 1-3% of the North American population. Although joint pain, swelling, and stiffness are the major symptoms, systemic involvement may include the following organ systems: skin, pulmonary, cardiac, neurologic, ophthalmologic, and hematopoietic. It is felt to be a disease of rather recent origin with Christopher Columbus, Mary Queen of Scots, and President James Madison being some of the more famous sufferers.

ETIOLOGY AND EPIDEMIOLOGY

Although the cause of RA is unknown, it is theorized that various infectious agents may incite the disease in genetically susceptible hosts. It has been recognized that 35% of patients with RA possess the Class II HLA-DR4 antigen present in only 13% of the normal Caucasian population. The fact that RA is a disease of primarily Caucasian people living in the temperate zones may be a reflection of the lower incidence of DR4 antigen in blacks and Asians who live in more tropical areas, or possibly of a geographic gradient in the distribution of some putative cause.

DIAGNOSIS

The diagnosis of RA is based primarily upon clinical findings. Criteria established by the American Rheumatism Association (ARA) in 1955 and revised in 1987 aid in making the diagnosis.

Table 26.1
Summary of the 1987 Revised Criteria for the Classification of Rheumatoid Arthritis

1. Morning stiffness in and around the joint, lasting at least one hour before maximal improvement.
2. Arthritis (soft tissues swelling or fluid) of three or more joint areas simultaneously and observed by a physician. The 14 possible bilateral areas are PIP, MCP, wrist, elbow, knee, ankle and MTP joints.
3. Arthritis of at least one area in a wrist, MCP, or PIP joint.
4. Symmetric arthritis (with simultaneous involvement).
5. Rheumatoid subcutaneous nodules over bony prominences, over extensor surfaces, or in juxtaarticular regions.
6. Serum rheumatoid factors (see Chapter 5).
7. Radiographic changes typical of RA on PA films of the hand and wrist.

A patient is said to have RA if at least 4 of these 7 criteria are met, and criteria 1-4 were present for a least 6 weeks (sensitivity 91-94% and specificity 89%).

COMPLICATIONS OF RA

Articular complications. Ongoing synovitis of the odonto-axial joint produces loosening and destruction of the odontoid and the ligament that keeps it in place with subsequent atlanto-axial subluxation and possible death from sudden movement of the neck.

Extra-articular complications. Although RA is a disease primarily affecting the joints, its systemic manifestation can be serious. Pleural involvement is the most common *pulmonary manifestation* but rarely compromises respiratory status. Bronchial disease is also common. Interstitial lung disease, seen more frequently in men with RA than in women, is present in 10-30% patients with RA. Symptoms consist primarily of dyspnea and a nonproductive cough. On rare occasions, it can cause severe hypoxemia and death. Radiographs show a reticulonodular infiltrate predominantly in the mid to lower lung fields. Histopathologically, the early changes are felt to be an inflammatory interstitial pneumonitis consisting of lymphocytes, plasma cells, and macrophages which later progresses to interstitial fibrosis. Although corticosteroids are usually given, many patients do not improve their respiratory status with treatment.

Pericarditis, another complication of RA, can be life-threatening. Evidence for pericarditis can be found in up to 50% of patients in some autopsy series, but only about 10% of patients have clinical evidence of pericarditis during this lifetime. Some patients with chronic pericarditis may respond to corticosteroids, while others, who develop tamponade or constrictive pericarditis, require pericardiectomy.

Rheumatoid vasculitis is one of the most serious complications of RA. Cutaneous, neurological, pulmonary, and GI involvement comprise the spectrum of this vasculitis. It involves primarily small arteries and venules, but medium-sized vessels can be involved. The etiology of vasculitis in RA is felt to be circulating immune complexes. Evidence supporting this is the presence of lower serum complement levels in RA patients with vasculitis than in those without, and the presence of immunoglobulin and complement deposited within involved vessel walls. The overall prognosis of rheumatoid vasculitis is unknown, but it is known that visceral infarction and presence of extensive motor neuropathy is associated with a poor prognosis. Treatment of rheumatoid vasculitis although not well studied, consists of corticosteroids with the addition of cyclophosphamide if patients do not respond to steroids alone.

Ophthalmologic complications of patients with RA include corneal involvement by keratoconjunctivitis sicca, episcleritis, and scleritis. Keratoconjunctivitis sicca or dry eyes is the most common eye complaint in RA patients. This manifestation of Sjögren's syndrome can cause corneal scarring and decreased visual acuity if ulcers and infections are allowed to develop. Scleritis can cause pain, thinning of the sclera, and ultimately perforation and blindness. (See Chapters 31 and 42.)

Secondary amyloidosis is a rare complication in patients with RA in the United States. Its incidence varies considerably, depending on whether the diagnosis is made clinically or on postmortem examination and whether the studies were done in North America or Europe. A 5% incidence of amyloidosis in adult RA patients is reported from Europe but appears much less frequently in the U.S.

Felty's syndrome is described as the classic triad of RA, splenomegaly, and granulocytopenia. Many RA patients with Felty's syndrome have rheumatoid nodules and other extra-articular manifestations of their disease such as vasculitis. Some patients with this syndrome suffer recurrent bacterial infections, while others remain free of infections. The level of the absolute granulocyte count does not correlate with risk of infection. In patients with recurrent life-threatening infections splenectomy may be life saving, but in some, it is of no use. Treatment with gold may be helpful in suppressing disease activity and allowing the granulocyte count to return to normal.

Adult onset Still's disease is an uncommon presentation in adults, consisting of intermittent, high, spiking fevers, an evanescent, salmon-colored, non-pruritic rash, and oligo- or polyarthritis. The wrists are characteristically involved and may develop ankylosis of the metacarpals and carpal bones. Sore throat, lymphadenopathy, pleuropericarditis, hepatosplenomegaly, and even amyloidosis have been reported. If other possible etiologies can be excluded and treatment with NSAIDs is unsatisfactory, steroids at a dose of 1 mg/kg may be required.

TREATMENT

Treatment of RA consists of an orderly progression of therapeutic steps beginning with salicylates (see also Chapters 43 through 48). Later therapy for more aggressive disease may involve more toxic medications such as the second line drugs or cytotoxic therapy. In select patients, low-dose daily steroids, or intermittent intra-articular or intravenous steroid boluses can be helpful.

Basic therapy consists of either salicylates or other non-steroidal anti-inflammatory medications plus physical (PT) and occupational therapy (OT). Educating patients about their disease is essential, even at early stages. Physical therapists teach range of motion exercises, use of ambulatory devices, and maintenance of muscle tone. These exercises should become part of the daily routine of patients with RA. Occupational therapists concentrate on the protection of the hand joints, use of splints, and adaptive devices. With significant hand and wrist involvement, attempts to maintain the most basic simple hygiene may become impossible for the patient. Adaptive devices can make a big difference.

If basic therapy fails to help, use of second line agents or cytotoxic drugs is instituted to protect joints from further damage and to maintain functional status (see Chapter 45). In general, these drugs do not exert a direct anti-inflammatory effect and are highly tissue bound. Hydroxychloroquine (an antimalarial drug) and gold salts (oral or parenteral forms) are the more commonly used second line drugs. D-penicillamine has been used as a second line agent for many years, but its popularity has declined due to its toxicity profile.

Among the cytotoxic drugs, azathioprine was the first approved by FDA for use by RA patients. It has achieved more widespread use in Canada than in the U.S. The antimetabolite, methotrexate, is now being used with increasing frequency because of its quick onset of action (3-4 weeks) and high rate of efficacy. It does not behave like a typical slow-acting drug, and it is thought that its primary effect is anti-inflammatory. Its long term toxicity is still being defined. Sulfasalazine, originally synthesized for RA, is now beginning to enjoy a resurgence in popularity as an additional second line drug. Decisions to progress from basic therapy to second line drugs or from one drug to another is based upon balancing side effects of medications with the patient's functional and anatomic status. The impact by these drugs on long-term prognosis of RA is probably limited. However, they clearly help delay the development of irreversible disability.

EVALUATING FUNCTIONAL CLASS

In 1949, Steinbrocker established criteria to assess functional status of patients with RA:

Class	*Definition*	*Remarks*
I	Capable of all activities	
II	Moderate restriction	Adequate for normal activities despite handicap or discomfort or limited motion at one or more joints
III	Marked restriction	Activity limited to self-care and few or no duties of a usual occupation
IV	Bed and/or chair confined	Capable of little or no self-care

Grades I and IV are particularly precise and useful, whereas Grades II and III contain large groups of patients with a wide spectrum of function within those classes.

RADIOGRAPHIC STAGING SYSTEM FOR RA

Stage	Definition
I	No destructive changes; periarticular osteopenia may be present.
II	Osteoporosis is definite, with or without slight subchondral bone destruction; slight joint space narrowing may be present.
III	Evidence for cartilage and bone destruction; joint deformity (e.g., subluxation, ulnar deviation) without bony or fibrous ankylosis.
IV	Stage III criteria plus fibrous or bony ankylosis.

From Steinbrocker O, et al. JAMA. 1949; 140:659-62.

An ideal response to a medication includes both improvement of functional class as well as prevention of joint destruction.

COMPLICATIONS OF TREATMENT

The most common side effects of *aspirin and nonsteroidal anti-inflammatory drugs* are gastric irritation and/or peptic ulcer formation, with or without overt bleeding, edema (which may worsen heart failure), and renal failure, especially in elderly dehydrated patients or patients with mild renal insufficiency. Rarely, one can see meningitis, hepatitis, or bone marrow suppression from some of these agents.

Side effects of second line agents can be more severe, e.g., nephrotic syndrome, exfoliative dermatitis, bone marrow aplasia, or acute pneumonitis. *D-penicillamine* rarely can cause immunologically-mediated diseases such as myasthenia gravis, poly/dermatomyositis, and lupus-like syndromes, Goodpasture's syndrome, bullous pemphigoid, and an obliterative alveolitis. (See Chapter 45 for specific side effects and how to monitor each drug.)

In patients who have been kept on daily steroids for any significant length of time, the ravages of iatrogenic Cushing's are likely to occur—osteopenia, thoracolumbar compression fractures, and fractures elsewhere, infections in prosthetic and natural joints, cataracts, etc. So while steroids may be life-saving or able to prolong gainful employment, the consequences can be dire, and patients who are placed on them should receive low doses (7.5 to 10 mg/day) for the least amount of time necessary.

PROGNOSIS

Although RA is primarily a chronic disabling disease, several studies have provided evidence that, in addition, it is associated with an increased mortality. In a prospective study in which RA patients were followed over 12 years, men with RA were four years younger at death than the median age of death in the general male population. Women with RA died 10 years earlier than the median age of death of the general female population. The two major causes of death were cardiovascular disease and malignancy, although there were some increased deaths due to sepsis and complications of rheumatoid disease like vasculitis, rheumatoid lung disease, and subluxation of the upper cervical spine. Some patients died from complications of arthritis therapy. Treatment with gold or prednisone did not affect survival.

PROBLEMS IN MANAGEMENT

Joint destruction is the ultimate result of uncontrolled synovitis. Over the past 10-20 years, many prosthetic joints have been developed which have revolutionized the surgical contribution to treatment of patients with RA. The knee and hip protheses have been particularly successful. They have transformed the lives of people who would otherwise have been wheelchair-bound or bedridden to productive members of society. The decision of when to do an arthroplasty is primarily based upon functional class and the amount of pain the patient has in the affected joint. The joint must also show significant damage radiographically.

Other less tangible problems in patients with RA include the stress of living with a chronic disease and dealing with daily pain. Surprisingly, secondary depression or other psychological disturbances occur in only about 7% of cases, less than in patients with primary fibromyalgia. However, secondary fibromyalgia is common in these patients because of their poor sleep from constant joint pain. In these patients, 10-25 mg of amitriptyline or doxepin q.h.s. can be very helpful.

For some patients, psychotherapy or biofeedback and relaxation techniques are of great benefit in improving the quality of life. The Arthritis Foundation offers classes in self-help and support groups which promote autonomy, better self-image, and improve function in daily life.

SUGGESTED READINGS

1. Arnett FC, Edworth SM, Bloch DA, et al. The American Rheumatism Association 1987 revised criteria for the classification of rheumatoid arthritis. Arthritis Rheum. 1988; 31:315-24.

2. Mitchell DM, Spitz PW, Young DY, et al. Survival, prognosis, and causes of death in rheumatoid arthritis. Arthritis Rheum. 1986; 29:706-714.

Chapter 27

Lupus Erythematosus

Systemic lupus erythematosus (SLE) is a multisystem disease of unknown etiology characterized by the presence of multiple auto-antibodies, some of which appear to participate in immunologically-mediated tissue injury. The diagnosis of systemic lupus erythematosus is based on: (1) the presence of multisystem disease, (2) the presence of auto-antibodies to cellular constituents, particular to nuclear components, and (3) the exclusion of other diseases. Because of the difficulty in establishing the diagnosis, the ARA devised and tested clinical and serologic criteria for the diagnosis. These criteria are listed below:

DIAGNOSIS OF SLE

The 1982 Revised Criteria for the Classification of Systemic Lupus Erythematosus

1. Malar or butterfly rash: fixed erythema, flat or raised over the malar eminences and sparing the nasolabial folds.
2. Discoid rash: erythematous raised patches of hyperkeratotic scaling and later atrophic scarring.
3. Photosensitivity described by the patient or observed by the physician.
4. Oral or nasopharyngeal ulcers that are usually painful.
5. Arthritis of two or more peripheral joints, traditionally non-erosive and non-deforming.
6. Serositis: pleuritis or pericarditis.
7. Renal disorder consisting of persistent proteinuria greater than 0.5 grams per day or presence of cellular casts in the urine.

8. Neurologic disorder in the form of seizures or psychoses unexplainable by other causes.
9. Hematologic abnormalities including autoimmune hemolytic anemia, leukopenia, or thrombocytopenia.
10. Immunologic disorder characterized by a positive LE cell preparation, or antibodies to double-stranded DNA, or antibodies to Sm nuclear antigen, or a false-positive serologic test for syphilis.
11. Antinuclear antibody positivity in the absence of drugs known to cause a positive ANA.

The presence of four or more criteria establishes the diagnosis of SLE with approximately 95% sensitivity and 96% specificity.

EPIDEMIOLOGY OF SYSTEMIC LUPUS ERYTHEMATOSUS

The incidence in the United States is 7.6 cases per 100,000 per year. Lupus affects all ages and both sexes, but it is predominantly a disease of young women with a peak incidence between the ages of 12 and 40. It is more frequent in black women ages 15 to 64, with a prevalence of one case per 254, while for all women in that same age group, the prevalence is one case per 700.

ETIOLOGY AND PATHOGENESIS

The etiology of systemic lupus erythematosus is unknown, but it appears to be multifactorial including a genetic predisposition, environmental factors, and putative viral agents. Lupus occurs in the relatives of lupus patients 100-200 times more frequently than in the general population, and there is an increased frequency of the HLA histocompatibility antigens DR_2 and DR_3. Hormonal factors also play a role. Lupus occurs more commonly in women in a ratio of 9:1 females to males. A number of studies have shown an increase in estrogen metabolites in both lupus patients and in their first degree relatives. An increased association of SLE with Klinefelter's syndrome has been reported with evidence of persistent estrogen stimulation in these men. Finally, there is a suggestion that oral contraceptive therapy may increase the risk of a flare in SLE patients.

The role of environmental factors in lupus is also unclear. Laboratory personnel and physicians who handle lupus sera reportedly have a greater frequency and concentration of antinuclear antibodies than do controls. It is thought that the major trigger of SLE is a virus although attempts at direct isolation of viruses and their by-products have been conflicting and unrewarding. The pathogenesis of lupus has been hypothesized as follows: a trigger, perhaps an unknown virus, in conjunction with genetic, hormonal, and environmental factors may cause a cascade of humoral and cellular immunodysregulation. In response to this trigger, B cells proliferate while T suppressor cell function decreases, leading to an increase in immunoglobulin-secreting cells. Production of multiple auto-antibodies is turned on, including antibodies to double-stranded DNA which appear to be pathogenetically involved in the production of inflammatory lupus nephritis. The circulating immune complexes of DNA and anti-DNA deposit in the glomerular basement membrane where complement is activated, resulting in tissue injury by the cellular mediators of inflammation.

ORGAN INVOLVEMENT IN SYSTEMIC LUPUS ERYTHEMATOSUS

1. *Skin*

   The most common form of skin involvement in SLE is a *malar rash* and/or a *photosensitive rash*. Two other more distinct syndromes may occur, subacute cutaneous lupus erythematosus (SCLE) or discoid lupus erythematosus (DLE).

   Discoid lupus erythematosus (DLE) is usually confined to the head and neck and begins with erythema and hyperpigmentation in a plaque-like appearance. As DLE continues, atrophy occurs in the center of the expanding plaque which although initially hyperpigmented becomes depigmented as it progresses. An important fact to remember about discoid lupus is that it is always scarring. If DLE is confined to the scalp, there is only a 10% chance that the patient will also have systemic involvement. In patients with SLE, however, 30% may have discoid lupus lesions.

   Subacute cutaneous lupus erythematosus (SCLE) usually involves photosensitive areas and is non-scarring, although it may result in areas of hyperpigmentation and telangiectasiae. Approximately 50% of people with subacute cutaneous lupus will satisfy criteria for systemic involvement.
2. *Kidney Involvement*

   In some reported series, the kidneys are involved in up to 50% of lupus patients, with severe renal involvement occurring in 25%. Renal involvement usually occurs within the first 1-2 years after the onset of SLE and is the second most common cause of death in SLE patients, after infection. The glomerulonephritis of SLE may be: (1) mesangial, (2) focal proliferative, (3) diffuse proliferative, or (4) membranous. Mesangial, focal, and diffuse proliferative glomerulonephritis appear to represent a continuum of inflammatory glomerular disease from benign to more aggressive involvement of the kidneys and will often respond to high-dose steroids and cytotoxic drugs. However, this view is not without controversy. Membranous nephropathy is noninflammatory and does not respond to steroids. A number of studies have suggested that the level of renal function and proteinuria may be as useful in determining prognosis as the histologic classification obtained from kidney biopsy. However, the chronic changes of glomerulosclerosis and/or tubulointerstitial fibrosis are more predictive of a poor outcome (either renal failure and/or renal death) than histologic classification alone.

The indications for a renal biopsy in SLE remain controversial. In a patient without clinical evidence of renal involvement, it is not indicated. If renal involvement is present at the time of diagnosis, or later, one may either biopsy or base initial treatment on the severity of the clinical manifestations with an empiric trial of high-dose steroids. Biopsy may be reserved for those patients who fail to improve substantially after a month of ongoing therapy.

3. *Pulmonary Manifestations*

Abnormal pulmonary function tests are common in asymptomatic SLE patients and are characterized by the presence of restrictive defects and/or a low diffusing capacity. Pleural effusions are seen in approximately 40% of SLE patients, and symptoms of pleuritis are even more common. Acute lupus pneumonitis is seen in less than 5% of patients. Its presentation is characterized by the sudden onset of dyspnea, fever, dry cough, and the presence of basilar infiltrates on chest x-ray. It is extremely important to rule out bacterial or fungal infections or drug toxicity in SLE patients who present in this fashion. When chronic, lupus pneumonitis is indistinguishable from idiopathic pulmonary fibrosis. Although pulmonary hemorrhage is uncommon, it may be massive and fatal and needs to be considered in the differential diagnosis of patients with lupus who present with acute dyspnea. Although hemoptysis may be present, suggesting the presence of pulmonary hemorrhage, it need not be.

4. *Cardiac Involvement*
Pericarditis with or without an effusion may be present but rarely leads to cardiac tamponade. Uncommonly, conduction abnormalities and coronary arteritis have also been described. Libman-Sacks verrucous endocarditis may be present at autopsy quite commonly but only rarely is clinically significant.
5. *Central Nervous System Manifestations*
Central nervous system manifestations are the most unpredictable and variable features of systemic lupus erythematosus. Psychoses and/or seizures are the most commonly reported findings, followed by cranial nerve palsies, major motor weakness, peripheral neuropathies, migraine headaches, chorea, transverse myelitis, and aseptic meningitis. There is no specific test to make the diagnosis of central nervous system lupus. It remains a diagnosis of exclusion. Oftentimes, the lumbar puncture, EEG, and CT scan are normal or nonspecific. Preliminary studies suggest that magnetic resonance imaging (MRI) may provide the necessary sensitivity to ascertain CNS involvement in SLE.
Anti-cardiolipin antibodies may be present in some patients with central nervous system manifestations, whereas others have antineuronal antibodies. What roles these antibodies have in the pathogenesis of CNS lupus remains uncertain. High dose corticosteroids to treat other manifestations of lupus may also result in manifestations mimicking CNS lupus, such as steroid psychosis. It must be considered in the differential diagnosis of these patients' symptoms.
6. *Other Clinical Features*
Hematologic manifestations include leukopenia, oftentimes associated with lymphopenia, thrombocytopenia (which is often autoimmune mediated) and a Coombs' positive hemolytic anemia. However, while Coombs' positivity occurs in approximately 25% of patients, hemolysis occurs in only 5%. Other clinical features include the presence of subcutaneous nodules in up to 10% of lupus patients.

LUPUS AND PREGNANCY

Young women with lupus who are pregnant are considered at high risk of fetal loss and maternal illness. Approximately 25% of lupus pregnancies result in a poor fetal outcome, characterized by spontaneous abortions or stillbirth. In addition, there is an increased incidence of intrauterine growth retardation and prematurity. Although uncommon, neonates may also develop either a permanent isolated heart block, thrombocytopenia, leukopenia, and/or rash consistent with subacute cutaneous lupus (neonatal lupus). Neonates of mothers with anti-SS-A antibodies in their serum are particularly at risk for this complication, although it is not the only risk factor. Although controversial, it appears lupus may flare either during or immediately after pregnancy.

DRUG-INDUCED SLE

Drug-induced lupus-like syndrome can be precipitated by the use of certain medications. The prototypes are procainamide and hydralazine. Patients with drug-induced lupus complain primarily of arthralgias and pleuropericardial symptoms with or without associated effusion. Central nervous system involvement and renal involvement do not occur in drug-induced lupus (although there have been occasional case reports). In addition, drug-induced lupus is associated with a much more restricted expression of autoantibody formation. Unlike systemic lupus, where multiple autoantibodies are found, drug-induced lupus is characterized by the presence of antibodies to single-stranded DNA and histones only. Antibodies to double-stranded DNA are absent.

PROGNOSIS AND TREATMENT

The overall prognosis of systemic lupus erythematosus has improved dramatically in the last 50 years with 10-year survival rates of 80-94%. There is no clear evidence that any one form of treatment is responsible for this improved prognosis. In fact, it is felt by some investigators that the disease itself has changed to a milder form although this is not completely substantiated. In addition, identification of earlier and milder cases may account for the apparent improvement in prognosis.

Treatment of systemic lupus erythematosus should be directed at the type and level of activity or organ system involvement. For example, aspirin and a variety of other nonsteroidal agents are excellent for managing lupus that primarily involves the joints and skin with constitutional symptoms. The anti-malarials, particularly chloroquine (Aralen) and hydroxychloroquine (Plaquenil) are also very beneficial in controlling skin and joint disease. The usual dose of Plaquenil is 200 mg b.i.d.

Corticosteroids in high dose should be reserved for those patients with potentially life-threatening central nervous system or renal involvement or with significant pleuropericardial or hematologic disease that has not responded to more conservative therapy.

Cutaneous involvement is best managed by avoidance of sun, proper use of sun screens (sun protection factor of 15 or more), and the use of antimalarials as needed. Autoimmune thrombocytopenia is traditionally treated with prednisone in a dose of 1-2 mg/kg/day with improvement in 50-75% of patients, usually within two weeks of therapy. The role of splenectomy in systemic lupus erythematosus is controversial. Newer forms of therapy for thrombocytopenia include the use of Danazol, a synthetic androgen, and intravenous gammaglobulin therapy.

Active lupus nephritis has been treated with high-dose oral prednisone in a dose of 1-2 mg/kg/day. IV pulse methylprednisolone at doses of 1 gm q.d. for two or three days has been used to obtain initial control of nephritis. Immunosuppressive therapy includes use of cyclophosphamide, azathioprine, or (more recently) methotrexate. Cyclophosphamide bolus therapy in a dose of 0.5-1 gm per M^2 per month shows promise of being beneficial with fewer toxic side effects than seen with oral daily cyclophosphamide therapy. Azathioprine has also been reported to be of benefit in some patients with lupus nephritis, and methotrexate is currently under investigation. Although severe central nervous system disease has been traditionally treated empirically with high dose corticosteroids, there is no good study to show benefit. In severe cases of central nervous system lupus, plasmapheresis and immunosuppressive agents are a last resort. In patients with thrombotic events, aspirin or anticoagulants have been used empirically.

Drug-induced lupus should be managed by stopping the causative drug. This is usually sufficient, although, with significant pleuropericardial disease, a short course of corticosteroids may be needed for symptomatic relief. The drug-induced ANA usually disappears within six months to a year after stopping the drug.

FINAL WORDS OF WISDOM ON THE MANAGEMENT OF SYSTEMIC LUPUS ERYTHEMATOSUS

1. Not all lupus patients require steroids. Mild disease, such as skin and joint involvement can often be well controlled with the use of non-steroidals and/or antimalarials.

2. If a lupus patient presents with fever, particularly if the patient is on high-dose steroids or on cytotoxic agents, infection *must* be the first consideration.
3. The only indications for immediate steroid therapy are life-threatening pulmonary hemorrhage, significant central nervous system disease, or bowel vasculitis. Lupus nephritis should be treated promptly in a few days but need not be treated emergently in a few hours.
4. Always remember to taper corticosteroids slowly in a patient with lupus in order to minimize both steroid withdrawal and reactivation of the underlying disease.
5. The main need in the medical management of a seriously ill patient with systemic lupus erythematosus is a capable, interested physician who is either an expert or has access to appropriate consultants with the necessary experience to help manage the patient's therapy.
6. An achy patient with a slight photosensitive rash and a positive ANA may or may not have SLE. This will become obvious over time. Do not commit her to steroids or cytotoxic drugs unless involvement of other organ systems warrants it. Do not make the diagnosis lightly, given the repercussions for life, health, disability insurance, and accompanying mental anguish.

SUGGESTED READINGS

1. Tan EM, Cohen AS, Fries JF, et al. The 1982 revised criteria for the classification of system lupus erythematosus. Arthritis Rheum. 1982; 25:1271-77.

2. Klippel JH, editor. Systemic lupus erythematosus. Rheum Dis Clin NA. 1988; 14:1-252.

Chapter 28

Systemic Sclerosis

The incidence of systemic sclerosis (scleroderma) is 20 cases per million population per year, an incidence higher than previously reported. Most scleroderma appears to be idiopathic, but scleroderma-like syndromes have been described in association with environmental and occupational hazards such as silica or vinyl chloride exposure, after cosmetic surgery such as breast augmentation with silicone implants, and with drug exposures, primarily the anti-cancer drug bleomycin, and the migraine prophylactic Sansert (methysergide). A localized type of sclerodermatous skin change can occur after repeated injections of pentazocine (Talwin). There was one unusual epidemic in Spain of an acute pulmonary febrile illness following ingestion of de-denatured rapeseed oil that evolved into a scleroderma-like syndrome in survivors.

DEFINITIONS

1. *Systemic sclerosis*: a generalized disorder of connective tissue characterized by inflammatory, fibrotic, and degenerative changes often accompanied by prominent vascular lesions in the skin, synovium and certain internal organs, notably the esophagus, intestinal tract, heart, lung, and kidney.
2. *Sclerodactyly*: thickening and atrophy of the skin proceeding distally from the metacarpophalangeal joints. Proximal scleroderma has similar changes proximal to the MCPs.
3. *Acrosclerosis*: sclerosis of the distal portion of the hands and feet.
4. *Morphea*: localized patches of scleroderma which tend to occur on the trunk and not distally. Progression to systemic involvement is rare.

5. *Linear scleroderma*: localized scleroderma in a linear fashion often involving deep structures usually seen in younger patients. It rarely crosses the midline or becomes systemic.
6. *Scleroderma* denotes the edematous, indurative and/or atrophic skin changes characteristically seen in progressive systemic sclerosis. These changes most often involve the hands, forearms, arms, face, and upper anterior chest, but also can involve the feet, legs, back, and abdomen. In addition, this term is used interchangeably with systemic sclerosis.
7. *Scleromyxedema*: widespread lichenoid plaques consisting of mucopolysaccharide deposition which is frequently associated with an IgM paraprotein.
8. *CREST syndrome*: the presence of calcinosis, Raynaud's phenomenon, esophageal dysmotility, sclerodactyly, and/or telangiectasias. This represents a milder subset of systemic sclerosis.

CLASSIFICATION

1. Systemic Sclerosis
   a. Diffuse Cutaneous Disease
      Onset of Raynaud's phenomenon within one year of skin changes
      Acral and truncal skin involvement
      Tendon friction rubs
      Early and severe involvement of lung (pulmonary fibrosis), kidneys (renal failure usually accompanied by accelerated hypertension), gastrointestinal, and/or myocardial disease
      Calcinosis 7%, telangiectasiae 50%
      Antibodies to Scl-70 in 25-30%
   b. Limited Cutaneous Disease ("CREST" syndrome)
      Raynaud's phenomenon often present for years before skin involvement
      Acral skin involvement
      Late appearance of pulmonary hypertension
      Calcinosis 40%, telangiectasiae 80%
      Anticentromere antibodies in 80%
   c. "Overlap" syndromes—in association with SLE, Sjögren's syndrome or polymyositis.
      Patients with features of SLE, scleroderma, myositis, and some-

times RA-like arthritis who have high titer antibodies to RNP and have a milder course than SLE with nephritis. This subgroup has been named Mixed Connective Tissue Disease (MCTD).

2. Localized Scleroderma
   a. morphea
   b. linear scleroderma
   c. "en coup de sabre"
3. Drug and environmental toxin related

PRELIMINARY CLINICAL CRITERIA FOR THE DIAGNOSIS OF SYSTEMIC SCLEROSIS

Proximal scleroderma is the single major criterion. The sensitivity of this criterion is 91% with a specificity of over 99%. Minor criteria are (1) sclerodactyly; (2) pitting scars of the fingertips or loss of substance of the distal finger pad; (3) bibasilar pulmonary fibrosis. One major or two or more minor criteria were found in 97% of definite scleroderma patients, but only 2% of patients with systemic lupus erythematosus, polymyositis, dermatomyositis, or Raynaud's phenomenon.

ORGAN SYSTEM INVOLVEMENT

Skin

Skin changes vary in extent and progression, dependent on whether the systemic sclerosis is of the limited or diffuse cutaneous type. Even more importantly, outcome differs. Diffuse disease is associated with rapidly progressive skin involvement and early susceptibility to joint contractures, and renal, cardiac, or pulmonary failure. Limited disease is mild in comparison, but with the potential for the late complications of pulmonary hypertension, malabsorption, and primary biliary cirrhosis.

Typical scleroderma skin changes occur in three phases: (a) the edematous phase which is characterized by non-pitting edema, often associated with severe pruritus and lasting one to three years; (b) thickening of the skin with a hide-bound appearance; and (c) atrophy, a late stage in which the dermis often softens generally except in the hands. Other skin manifestations attributable to systemic sclerosis include:

a. digital pitting scars or loss of substance from the finger pad which appear as depressed areas at the tips of the digits, or loss of digital

Table 28.1.
Classification of Raynaud's Phenomenon

Primary: Without clinically apparent underlying disease, affects young women (often with a positive family history), no digital pitting.

Secondary:

1. Associated with a connective tissue disease (CTD)

CTD	% with Raynaud's
Scleroderma	90-95
MCTD	80-85
SLE	15-25
DM-PM	5-10
RA	5
JRA	rare
Vasculitis	rare

2. Associated with hyperviscosity—e.g., cryoproteins, polycythemia rubra vera, etc.
3. Arterial occlusive disease—e.g., Buerger's disease
4. Trauma—occupationally related blood vessel injury e.g., pneumatic hammer use
5. Thoracic outlet syndrome
6. Drugs and toxins—e.g., vinyl chloride, bleomycin, ergots, amphetamines, beta blockers
7. Reflex sympathetic dystrophy

pad tissue from ischemia rather than trauma or other exogenous causes;

b. bilateral finger or hand edema: firm non-pitting edema especially involving the fingers (includes puffy, sausage-like swelling of the fingers) over the dorsal aspects of the hands;
c. abnormal skin pigmentation with areas of hyperpigmentation or depigmentation ("pepper and salt");
d. telangiectasias: visible macular dilatation of superficial blood vessels which collapse upon pressure and fill slowly when pressure is released; distinguished from rapidly filling spider angioma with a central arterial feeding vessel and from dilated linear superficial veins. The periungual capillaries also experience changes with loss of some capillaries and telangiectatic dilatation of others. These changes are usually obvious to the naked eye but are best seen with a magnifying lens. Some investigators believe that marked abnor-

mality of periungual capillaries may be predictive of internal organ involvement;

e. Raynaud's phenomenon: at least a two-phase color change in the fingers and often toes consisting of pallor, cyanosis, and/or reactive hyperemia in response to cold exposure or emotion as determined by the patient's history and the physician's observation. A classification of Raynaud's phenomenon is shown below.

Lungs. Pulmonary involvement in scleroderma includes:

a. Bibasilar pulmonary fibrosis with a bilateral reticular pattern of linear or lineo-nodular densities which are most pronounced in the basilar portions of the lungs on standard chest radiographs. The pulmonary fibrosis may assume the appearance of diffuse mottling or "honey-comb lung" (associated with anti-Scl-70 antibody);
b. pulmonary hypertension which may be due to obliterative vasculopathy as seen in the CREST variety of scleroderma or may be secondary to scleroderma parenchymal disease with extensive pulmonary fibrosis;
c. vascular reactivity to cold;
d. It should also be noted that there appears to be an increased frequency of bronchoalveolar carcinoma in late-stage scleroderma lung disease, even in non-smokers.

Gastrointestinal Tract. Gastrointestinal manifestations include:

a. lower (distal) esophageal dysphagia characterized by substernal discomfort on swallowing or the sensation of food sticking in the retrosternal location;
b. lower (distal) esophageal dysmotility with hypoperistalsis or aperistalsis as demonstrated by either cine-esophagogram, fluoroscopy, or by manometric study. This is often accompanied by evidence of decreased lower esophageal sphincter tone with reflux of the gastric contents into the esophagus;
c. colonic sacculations consisting of wide-mouthed diverticuli of the colon located along the anti-mesenteric border, found on barium enema examination; these sacculations may also occur in the ileum and jejunum. With long-standing disease, bacterial overgrowth in the hypotonic bowel is associated with malabsorption which may be profound but is treatable with oral antibiotics every few weeks. Long-standing scleroderma bowel has been has been successfully managed by intravenous hyperalimentation at home.

Heart. Cardiac manifestations include:

a. pericarditis with or without an associated effusion. The presence of a pericardial effusion is often the harbinger of renal disease within three to six months of its appearance;

b. cardiomegaly with congestive heart failure;
c. cardiomegaly with conduction defects or nodal or ventricular arrhythmias.

Musculoskeletal System. Musculoskeletal manifestations include:

a. articular complaints: 90% of patients with scleroderma will complain of arthralgias. A much fewer number complain of definite inflammation or swelling of one or more joints and/or tenosynovitis. Tendon and/or joint creaking due to fibrin deposition may also occur in diffuse scleroderma;
b. muscle weakness and/or pain with or without other findings of myositis;
c. bone involvement may include resorption of digital tufts, the radius, ulna, clavicle, jaw or ribs, generally in association with soft tissue calcifications (calcinosis).

Kidneys. Renal manifestations occur almost exclusively in diffuse scleroderma and include:

a. proteinuria in excess of 3.5 grams/24 hours;
b. persistent excessive cellular casts in the urinary sediment;
c. creatinine clearance less than 45 cc/minute and
d. rapidly progressive renal failure. Patients with renal involvement from diffuse systemic sclerosis have the highest mortality. These patients often present with the rapid onset of high renin hypertension, often without proteinuria at the time of presentation. Normotensive scleroderma renal crisis may also occur infrequently. Predictors of patients who might develop kidney involvement include rapid progression of skin disease and pericardial effusion.

ETIOLOGY AND PATHOGENESIS

The etiology of scleroderma is unknown but the pathogenesis appears to involve both vascular injury and immunologic mechanisms.

LABORATORY FEATURES OF SCLERODERMA

Until recently, it was reported that antinuclear antibodies occurred in 25-70% of patients with scleroderma with the lower figure being more generally accepted. This was taken to imply that immunological abnormalities were not as prominent a feature in scleroderma as in other connective tissue diseases such as systemic lupus erythematosus and Sjögren's syndrome. More recently, the use of human tissue culture cells as substrate for the ANA test has led to a notable increase in the frequency of ANA positivity. A positive ANA is now found in over 95% of patients with scleroderma. There are a number of more specific autoantibodies that have been reported in systemic sclerosis that include antibodies to Scl-70 (a marker for diffuse disease) in 25%, anti-RNP in 20-30%, anti-centromere in 33%, and antinucleolar antibodies. In patients with CREST, over 90% exhibit antibodies to centromere in their sera. In contrast, only 3-10% of patients with diffuse scleroderma will have anticentromere antibodies.

General laboratory studies are normal unless the patient has significant renal disease or malabsorption. Microangiopathic hemolytic anemia may occur in the setting of scleroderma renal crisis, and is diagnosed by the characteristic morphologic changes of the red cells on the peripheral smear.

PROGNOSIS

In diffuse disease, the most common causes of death include scleroderma renal disease, heart or lung involvement, and starvation due to malnutrition. Patients with limited disease have a much better life expectancy but with the potential late complication of pulmonary hypertension.

TREATMENT OF SCLERODERMA

The only therapy that has made any long-term difference in mortality from PSS is aggressive, early treatment of hypertension. Even "borderline hypertension" in these patients should be treated aggressively with diastolic pressures in the 70s being a good target.

Otherwise, there is no specific treatment which has been shown to impact significantly on the course of scleroderma, with the possible exception of penicillamine, which may delay or prevent progression of major organ involvement. Penicillamine disrupts the cross-linking of collagen and may be useful in some patients but requires extended therapy to be efficacious. If penicillamine is to be used, it should be in a "go low-go slow" approach starting with 250 mg/day and gradually increasing over weeks to months to 750 mg/day. The basis for this recommendation is retrospective studies in non-randomized patients. We are all awaiting the results of prospective randomized trials.

Looking specifically at treatments tried in scleroderma:

a. corticosteroids are useful only for significant arthritis and/or myositis and do not appear to impact favorably on the skin disease;
b. immunosuppressive agents appear to be useful only for the arthritis and/or the myositis;
c. colchicine, which has been used because of its apparent effect in stimulating collagenase, may be useful for the skin although this is controversial and there appear to be no favorable effects on sclerosis of the internal organs;
d. coumadin appears not to be useful in treating calcinosis;
e. total lymphoid irradiation: preliminary studies suggest that it is not helpful or useful. It is strictly experimental.

Symptomatic treatment includes the use of cimetidine 400 mg q.i.d. or other H-2 blockers in the treatment of *reflux esophagitis*. Reglan in a dose of 10 mg at bedtime also provides symptomatic relief. Malabsorption due to bacterial overgrowth can be treated empirically with antibiotics (Flagyl 250 mgs t.i.d. and Keflex 250 mg q.i.d. for 7-10 days every few weeks).

As mentioned above, the *hypertension* associated with scleroderma renal crisis appears to respond favorably to vigorous antihypertensive therapy, particularly with angiotensin-converting enzyme inhibitors such as captopril and enalapril. For *severe renal disease*, hemodialysis and/or transplantation may be required. *Raynaud's* phenomenon is best treated by avoidance of provocative factors such as cold exposure. Various vasodilating calcium blockers have all been used with varying degrees of success. This is not surprising, since the vascular component of scleroderma is structural as well as vasospastic. If calcium channel blockers are used, verapamil should be tried last because of its ability to induce block through the AV node and the risk of associated arrhythmias.

SUGGESTED READINGS

1. LeRoy EC, Black C, Fleischmajer R, et al. Scleroderma (systemic sclerosis): Classification, subsets and pathogenesis. J. Rheumatol. 1988; 15: 202-205

2. Owens GR, Medsger TA Jr. Systemic sclerosis secondary to occupational exposure. Am J Med. 1988; 85:114-16.

3. Medsger TA Jr. Treatment of systemic sclerosis. Rheum Dis Clin North Am. 1989; 15:513-31.

Chapter 29

Weakness as a Presenting Complaint

Weakness, diminished strength of muscle contraction, results in loss of motor function. Although it seems to be a simple concept, patients often find it difficult to describe their complaint. They may use vague, descriptive terms such as fatigue, deadness, tiredness, or achiness. Because weakness has so many different etiologies, the importance of taking a careful history cannot be underestimated. Points to be covered when taking the history include:

family history of similar disease,
difficulty keeping the eyes open,
intermittent changes in the voice,
change in facial appearance,
presence of dysphagia, atrophy, fasciculations, cramps,
proximal or distal weakness,
sensory changes,
bowel or bladder dysfunction, and
change in functional status.

Establishing whether the weakness is brought on by exercise or is present regardless, and whether it resolves quickly or not is also useful.

The causes of weakness can be classified into two broad categories of upper motor neuron and lower motor neuron disease. Upper motor neuron disease refers to deficits either in the cerebral hemispheres, brainstem, or spinal cord. Lower motor neuron disease includes abnormalities of the anterior horn cell of the spinal cord, nerve root, peripheral nerve, neuromuscular junction, or muscle.

Patients with peripheral neuropathy often have predominantly distal weakness, paresthesias, and numbness.

Patients with myelopathy, in addition to weakness, have loss of bowel and bladder control. Examination of such patients may reveal fasciculations, hyperactive deep tendon reflexes, sensory changes, or presence of other upper motor neuron signs together with lower motor neuron signs at the level of myelopathy.

Patients with disorders of the neuromuscular junction usually have myasthenia gravis, Eaton-Lambert syndrome, or drug-induced myopathy.

Patients with myopathy usually have the gradual onset of symmetrical, proximal weakness with preservation of deep tendon reflexes. Although muscle pain can occur with myopathy, it is usually not severe. Once weakness has been determined to be of myopathic origin, it can be further divided into inherited myopathies, those associated with endocrine disorders, or a large group of acquired myopathies secondary to infections, toxins (drugs), or unknown etiology.

CLASSIFICATION OF MYOPATHIES

I. Inherited myopathies
   A. Muscular dystrophies
      1. X-linked Duchenne's
      2. Fascio-scapulo-humeral
      3. Limb-girdle
      4. Ocular
      5. Others
   B. Malignant hyperthermia
   C. Glycogen storage diseases, e.g., McArdle's disease (muscle phosphorylase deficiency)
   D. Congenital myopathy, e.g., Nemaline—rod, central core, etc.
   E. Myotonia
   F. Periodic paralysis—hyper-, hypo-, or normo-kalemic paralysis

II. Myopathies associated with endocrine disorders
   A. Hyperthyroidism/hypothyroidism
   B. Hyperadrenalism—Cushing's syndrome
   C. Acromegaly
   D. Hyper/hypoparathyroidism
   E. Primary aldosteronism with hypokalemia

III. Acquired Myopathies
- A. Infectious
  1. Viral—coxsackie, adeno, influenza A and B, parainfluenza, Epstein-Barr virus, ECHO, HTLV-1, HIV, etc.
  2. Bacterial—streptococcal, staphylococcal, Yersinia, leprosy, etc.
  3. Fungal—Candida, etc.
  4. Parasitic—trichinosis, toxoplasmosis, amoebiasis, cysticercosis, etc.
- B. Idiopathic
  1. Typical polymyositis (represents 35-60% of inflammatory myopathies)
  2. Typical dermatomyositis
  3. Dermatomyositis associated with malignancy
  4. Childhood dermatomyositis
  5. Polymyositis associated with connective tissue diseases
- C. Associated with diseases of unknown etiology
  1. Sarcoidosis
  2. Inclusion body myositis
  3. Granulomatous myositis
  4. Eosinophilic myositis (some are due to L-tryptophan)
- D. Toxins/Drugs
  1. Alcohol
  2. Corticosteroids
  3. Vincristine
  4. Clofibrate
  5. Chloroquine
  6. Colchicine
  7. Amodiaquine
  8. Penicillamine
  9. Lovastatin (in combination with other drugs)
  10. And many others

DIAGNOSTIC TESTS

The following tests are used most often in diagnosing patients with myopathy.

a. Elevation of the muscle enzymes *creatine kinase* (CK) and *aldolase* are commonly seen in patients with myopathies. This may be due either to muscle enzyme leak or muscle necrosis. The CK enzyme exists in three isoenzymic forms. The MM form predominates in cardiac and skeletal muscle, the MB form in cardiac muscle, and the BB isoenzyme is the major type present in the brain and smooth muscle. Although CK is useful to follow the course of the disease and response to therapy, this enzyme can become elevated with strenuous exercise, minor injuries to muscle, or very sustained muscular activity, so it is not very specific. In addition, well relatives of dystrophy patients have elevated CKs if they are carriers of the gene.

b. Other laboratory tests indicating muscle injury or myopathy include *myoglobinemia* and *myoglobinuria*, and *creatinuria*. Excessive creatinuria results from diseased muscles and from neuromuscular disorders that produce atrophy of muscle.

c. The *electromyogram* (EMG) is useful to distinguish between myopathies and diseases of the nervous system. In patients with myopathies, one sees abnormal electrical activity characterized by short duration, small, low amplitude, polyphasic potentials, At rest, the muscles of patients with myopathy produce no electrical activity with the exception of patients with polymyositis where fibrillation or muscle irritability can be seen. Late in the disease, the EMG is not helpful in determining activity of the myopathy.

d. A muscle biopsy is often done to confirm the presence of myopathy and to determine the exact type of myopathy present. The muscle selected for biopsy should be weak and actively involved by the disease process but not severely wasted. If possible, the side opposite from that studied by EMG is chosen to avoid false positive results from biopsying the EMG needle track. Histochemical staining of the muscle is done in addition to routine H & E stains. The former technique distinguishes muscle fiber types:

   Type 1 fibers are rich in oxidative enzymes and mitochondria, and

   Type 2 fibers are rich in myofibrillar ATPase and phosphorylase.

   An example of the utility of histochemical staining is seen in the myopathy of patients with disuse atrophy and long-term corticosteroid use, which is characterized by atrophy of type 2 fibers. In myopathic diseases, such as polymyositis, the characteristic pathologic findings are muscle necrosis, phagocytosis, regeneration, and perifascicular atrophy involving both fiber types. In addition, chronic inflammatory cells, located in the perivascular areas, are commonly seen in polymyositis and dermatomyositis.

   It is important to remember that many patients are unable to determine if weakness or pain is limiting the use of their muscles. Severe pain is rarely seen in myopathic diseases but may be present early in the course of acute onset polymyositis. Therefore, if pain is the predominant symptom, other diseases, not myopathies, are likely to be causing it. These diseases include polymyalgia rheumatica, proximal joint involvement by rheumatoid arthritis or other inflammatory arthritides, radicular pain and weakness, or fibromyalgia.

SUGGESTED READINGS

1. Mastaglia FL, Ojeda VJ. Inflammatory myopathies: Part 1 and 2. Annals of Neurology. 1985: 17:215-227.

2. Kagen LJ. Approach to the patient with myopathy. Bull Rheum Dis. 1983; 33(2):1-8.

3. Carpenter S, Karpati G, et al. Inclusion body myositis: A distinct variety of idiopathic inflammatory myopathy. Neurology. 1978; 28:8-17.

Chapter 30

Polymyositis and Dermatomyositis

Polymyositis (PM) and dermatomyositis (DM) are acquired, idiopathic inflammatory myopathies which can affect people of all ages. Although the highest incidence is in women in the 4th to 6th decades of life, the female predominance is particularly marked in a subset of patients who have associated connective tissue diseases such as systemic lupus erythematosus or scleroderma. Only in PM/DM of childhood is there a male predominance.

CLINICAL PRESENTATION

The most common presenting symptom of these diseases is the insidious onset of weakness involving the proximal muscle groups of the extremities. Pain, although uncommon, may occur with extensive muscle damage. Other muscle groups often involved include the pharyngeal muscles with can lead to aspiration pneumonia, and the myocardium, which can be a rare cause of death in these patients. Systemic features can include interstitial lung disease and vasculopathy. Vascular abnormalities seen are endothelial proliferation of the vessel, often with resultant occlusion of the lumen. True vasculitis with inflammatory cells within the vessel walls is not seen in these diseases. However, a characteristic periungual erythema from dilatation of these capillaries may be seen.

DIFFERENTIAL DIAGNOSIS

PM/DM must be distinguished from other myopathies as well as from proximal neuropathies. The following conditions should be excluded before making a diagnosis of idiopathic inflammatory myositis.

1. Evidence of central or peripheral neurologic disease
2. Muscular dystrophy
3. Preceding viral infection
4. Myasthenia gravis
5. Endocrinopathies such as hyper- or hypothyroidism, Cushing's syndrome, hyperparathyroidism, or hypoparathyroidism
6. Drugs and toxin exposure (alcohol, clofibrate, penicillamine, chloroquine, colchicine, etc.). Most recently eosinophilic myositis was described 2° to L-tryptophan ingestion.
7. Infectious myopathies (trichinosis, schistosomiasis, trypanosomiasis, staphylococcal, toxoplasmosis, HTLV-1, HIV, etc.)
8. Metabolic disorders such as McArdle's syndrome and other glycogen-storage diseases
9. Rhabdomyolysis
10. Granulomatous myositis

ETIOLOGY

Although the etiology of PM/DM is unknown, it is recognized that certain infectious agents can cause myositis. These organisms include viruses such as coxsackie, adeno, influenza, parainfluenza, and Epstein-Barr as well as bacteria such as *Streptococcus, Staphylococcus, Yersinia,* and leprosy. Lastly, parasites such as Trichinella, and Cysticercus have been implicated as causative agents of myositis. Some patients diagnosed with PM have serological evidence of recent infections with *Toxoplasma gondii*. In Jamaica, most patients with PM were shown to have HTLV-1 infection. In most patients with myositis, however, no specific infectious etiology is discovered. Although antimyosin antibodies have been demonstrated in some patients with PM/DM (predominantly in pediatric cases), most people believe cellular immunity with lymphocytoxicity against muscle plays a more important role than serologic immunity. Vasculopathy without vasculitis is seen in some muscle biopsies from children and has been associated with a poorer prognosis and even death.

DIAGNOSIS: (also see Chapter 29 on weakness)

In 1975, Bohan and Peter defined five criteria to diagnoses PM/DM, based on the physical findings and laboratory and histopathologic findings.

1. Symmetrical weakness of limb-girdle muscles and anterior neck flexors.

2. Muscle biopsy evidence of necrosis of Type I and II fibers, phagocytosis, regeneration, and basophilia, often with an inflammatory infiltrate with lymphocytes predominating.
3. Elevation in serum of skeletal muscle enzymes, particularly creatine kinase (CK), aldolase, and transaminases.
4. Electromyographic findings of short, small, polyphasic motor units, fibrillations, positive sharp waves, and insertional irritability.
5. Dermatologic features: heliotrope and Gottron's sign (flat, violaceous papules over the knuckles).

Although each criterion is *not* specific for PM/DM, the combination of three or four provides reasonable confidence levels in making the diagnosis.

CLASSIFICATIONS

PM/DM were classified by Bohan and Peter into five groups listed below. The percent of each subgroup in their series is thought to be representative of the population at referral centers.

Group I	Primary polymyositis (34%)
Group II	Primary dermatomyositis (29%)
Group III	Dermatomyositis or polymyositis associated with neoplasia (8.5%)
Group IV	Childhood dermatomyositis (7.5%)
Group V	Polymyositis or dermatomyositis with an associated "collagen vascular" disease (21%)

COMPLICATIONS OF THE DISEASE

An area of great controversy is the question of increased risk of malignancy in patients with these diseases. The risk is reported to be highest in men over the age of 50 who present with dermatomyositis. Unfortunately, early reports of increased incidence of malignancy are now felt to be exaggerated because patients with neuromuscular syndromes other than documented PM/DM were included. It is presently recommended that a complete history and physical examination be done in addition to routine surveillance blood work, chest x-ray, stool guaiacs, and urinalysis. In a woman, mammography should also be done. If any abnormality is found, further investigation is indicated. A more extensive malignancy work-up is unlikely to be of benefit. Although any neoplasm can be associated with these illnesses, the most commonly reported ones are lung, ovary, stomach, and breast.

Another complication of these diseases is aspiration pneumonia which can occur in patients with weak pharyngeal muscles. If patients show evidence of aspiration, feeding through a Dobhoff tube early in the course of treatment may be necessary. The normal swallowing mechanisms usually return several months after institution of treatment.

Calcinosis of muscle and skin occurs rarely (and mostly in children). When it does occur, contractures of muscles and skin result in severe functional disability for the patient.

TREATMENT

Corticosteroids are the mainstay of polymyositis and dermatomyositis therapy although there are no controlled studies reported confirming their efficacy. Prednisone is usually begun at 1 mg/kg in divided doses for the first two to three weeks. The dose is then consolidated into one daily dose. Steroids are slowly tapered (5 mg/week for the next few months) when muscle enzymes return to normal. Muscle strength returns slowly several months after the enzymes normalize. Steroid taper should be done more slowly (2.5 mg/1-2 weeks) once the daily steroid dose is less than 20 to 30 mg/day.

If patients fail to respond to steroids, are unable to be weaned off high doses, or have unacceptable side effects, immunosuppressive drugs, especially methotrexate and azathioprine are recommended. In uncontrolled studies in which methotrexate was used, a steroid-sparing effect and clinical response in 77% of patients was observed. In a controlled study of combined prednisone and azathioprine versus prednisone alone, at the end of one year patients receiving combined therapy showed significant benefit and were able to reduce the dose of prednisone. Other modalities, such as plasmapheresis in combination with immunosuppressives or intravenous serum globulin therapy have been tried and felt to be beneficial in some patients in uncontrolled trails.

Once acute inflammation in the muscle has subsided as determined by normalization of the muscle enzymes, a program of active physical therapy should be instituted. This is done to strengthen muscles and to maintain normal range of motion. Even during the acute stage of the disease, passive range of motion should be undertaken to prevent contractures.

Lack of response to steroids and cytotoxic medications suggests a rare disease, *inclusion body myositis*. This form of myositis is seen predominantly in males, most often has a benign course, and tends to involve distal more than proximal muscles.

COMPLICATIONS OF THERAPY

The major risk of treatment with corticosteroids and immunosuppressives is an increased incidence of infections. Patients should be monitored carefully for side effects from these medications, which include bone marrow suppression and liver toxicity.

Steroid myopathy, resulting from too high a dose of steroids, can occasionally cause weakness in the thigh and arm muscles. Normal muscle enzymes and improvement in muscle strength as the steroid dose is tapered help to differentiate between steroid myopathy and active myositis. On rare occasions, a muscle biopsy is needed to differentiate between the two. In steroid myopathy, one sees only Type 2-B atrophy without any inflammatory cells. In addition, finding an elevated urine creatine level in the presence of normal muscle enzymes is said to be suggestive of steroid myopathy.

PROGNOSIS

The natural history of these diseases is not well known or studied, due, in part, to most patients being treated with steroids. However, an uncontrolled study from 1963 showed that 23% of patients got significantly better or went into remission on their own without medication, which was not significantly different from patients treated with either low or high dose steroids. Of 26 of the patients in this study who died, deaths were fairly equally distributed among patients treated with high dose or low dose steroids or none at all. Criticisms of this study are that it was done retrospectively, and diagnostic criteria were not rigidly applied. More recent studies of survival of treated patients with adult PM/DM show eight-year survival rates of 73%, with patients less than 45 years of age at the time of diagnosis having the best prognosis.

SUGGESTED READINGS

1. Bohan A, Peter J. Polymyositis and dermatomyositis. N Engl J Med. 1975; 292:344-47, 403-07.

2. Hochberg MC, et al. Adult onset polymyositis/dermatomyositis: An analysis of clinical and laboratory features and survival in 76 patients with a review of the literature. Sem Arthritis Rheum. 1986; 15:168-78.

3. Metzger AL, Bohan A, Goldberg LS, et al. Polymyositis and dermatomyositis: Combined methotrexate and corticosteroid therapy. Ann Intern Med. 1974; 81:182-89.

4. Plotz, PH, Dalakas M, Leff RL, Love LA, Miller FW, Cronin ME. Current concepts in the idiopathic inflammatory myopathies: Polymyositis, dermatomyositis and related disorders. Ann Intern Med. 1989; 111:143-57.

Chapter 31

Keratoconjunctivitis Sicca, Xerostomia, and Sjögren's Syndrome

Dry eyes (keratoconjunctivitis sicca or KCS) and dry mouth (xerostomia) are common clinical findings, especially in the elderly. Several epidemiologic studies have reported a prevalence of dry eyes in this age group of 10% and higher. In this population, these symptoms are often secondary to various medications the patients may be taking rather than to a systemic rheumatic disease.

Because of the difficulty in defining the syndrome, investigators in Denmark, Japan, Greece, and the United States have proposed diagnostic criteria for primary Sjögren's syndrome (SS). The criteria we favor are those developed at the Scripps Clinic in San Diego, California. They are based on objective findings and clearly identify the features of autoimmunity which we have come to expect in patients with KCS, xerostomia, and typical lymphocytic infiltrates of the salivary glands diagnosed as primary Sjögren's syndrome.

Swelling and tenderness of salivary glands in association with dry mouth and enlargement of the lacrimal glands was first described by Mikulicz in 1892. In 1933, Henrik Sjögren described the association of dry mouth, dry eyes, and chronic deforming arthritis. In the 1950s, Morgan and Castleman went further by defining a subset of patients with dry eyes and dry mouth who had a systemic autoimmune disease. Since then, the heterogeneity of patients with these symptoms has come to be appreciated.

SCRIPPS CLINIC DIAGNOSTIC CRITERIA FOR SS

A. Inclusion criteria:
   1. Keratoconjunctivitis
      a. Decreased tear flow rate demonstrated by an abnormal Schirmer's test. This is done by inserting a strip of filter paper between the unanesthetized inferior palpebral and bulbar conjunctivae and measuring the extent ot wetting of the filter paper at 5 minutes. Normally it should be 10 or more millimeters. The results may vary with the temperature and humidity of the room and other factors.
      b. Increased staining of the corneal epithelium with rose bengal or fluorescein dye. The staining pattern is usually characteristic and consists of punctate staining that is more intense in the area of the palpebral aperture. The test is more sensitive when done with rose bengal.
   2. Xerostomia that is symptomatic and accompanied by decreased basal and stimulated salivary flow rate. Clinically, this manifests as absent pool of saliva under the tongue. Stimulation of flow can be done with lemon juice, and various tests have been advocated to measure salivary flow. Each of these tests have advantages and disadvantages. No one test has emerged as best.
   3. Lymphocytic infiltration of minor salivary glands demonstrated on lip biopsy obtained through normal mucosa. This has traditionally been considered a less morbid procedure than parotid gland biopsy, and specific findings have been advocated to diagnose SS. However, a recent report compared the sensitivity of lower lip biopsy with biopsy of the parotid gland via a postauricular approach and found that the parotid gland biopsy was 100% sensitive as opposed to 58% for the labial biopsy. It was also more specific than the lip biopsy. In addition, in the expert hands of the investigators, there was no morbidity from parotid gland biopsy but some minor morbidity from lip biopsy. (However, the usual practice still is to perform lip biopsy).
   4. Laboratory evidence of autoimmunity demonstrated by a positive rheumatoid factor of 1:160 or greater, or positive antinuclear antibody of 1:160 or greater, or positive SS-A or SS-B antibody.

B. Exclusion criteria
   1. Pre-existing lymphoma
   2. Graft versus host disease
   3. Acquired immunodeficiency disease (AIDS)
   4. Sarcoidosis

A *definite* diagnosis is made when all four criteria and exclusions are met. *Possible* SS is diagnosed if only three of the criteria are present.

FINDINGS ASSOCIATED WITH PRIMARY SS

In addition to the findings of KCS and xerostomia, extraglandular involvement is common in primary SS. Arthralgias, arthritis, thyroiditis, nephritis, anemia, pneumonitis, and interstitial pulmonary fibrosis, pulmonary hypertension, hyperglobulinemia, purpura, pleural effusions, myalgias, vasculitis and vasculopathy, neuropathies, and central nervous system involvement with various clinical manifestations have all been described. Vaginal dryness and dyspareunia are also common in women with this syndrome.

Less common but reported associations are celiac sprue and cholangitis. Patients with primary SS are at increased risk of developing non-Hodgkin's lymphoma, and this risk is increased several fold after receiving cytotoxic drugs. Pseudo-lymphoma has also been described and is considered by some as part of the spectrum between benign and malignant proliferation of lymphocytes in Sjögren's syndrome.

THE TEAR FILM

In addition to the abnormalities in the tear film seen in KCS from *aqueous* (or middle) layer deficiency, the two other layers of the tear film may be abnormal and produce symptoms similar to those seen in KCS.

Low intake of vitamin A produces an abnormal *mucin* layer unable to function as the wetting agent that adheres the aqueous layer to the anterior globe. This condition is readily identified by experienced ophthalmologists as xerosis and, when severe, produces typical small, gray, foamy plaques (Bitot spots). Classically, these patients first present with night blindness.

An abnormal *lipid* (the outermost) layer from hydrolysis of lipids by bacterial lipases and excessive release of free fatty acids occurs in blepharitis and can also produce symptoms of KCS. Blepharitis is a much more common condition than KCS and responds to local care. This condition can be excluded by an ophthalmologic examination.

OTHER CAUSES OF DRY EYES AND DRY MOUTH AND/OR ENLARGEMENT OF THE SALIVARY GLANDS

1. Anxiety.
2. Viral infection with Epstein-Barr virus, mumps, coxsackie A, ECHO virus, lymphocytic choriomeningitis, and human immunodeficiency virus (HIV-1).
3. Bacterial (involvement of the parotids is almost always due to *Staphyloccus aureus*), mycobacterial (tuberculous), or fungal (usually actinomyces) infections.
4. Local disease—mostly neoplasia or stones.
5. Systemic conditions like sarcoidosis, pemphigoid, amyloidosis, diabetes, pancreatitis, cirrhosis, lymphoma, and hyperlipidemias (Types II, IV, V).
6. Dietary factors and medications—alcoholism, malnutrition, anorexia, bulimia, iodides, anticholinergics, beta blockers, antihistamines, tranquilizers, antiparkinsonian drugs, and radiation therapy. Artificial tears with preservatives when used more often than every 2-3 hours may destabilize the tear film and actually worsen symptoms of dry eyes.

APPROACH TO THE TREATMENT OF PATIENTS WITH DRY EYES AND DRY MOUTH

Patients are likely to present to ophthalmologists complaining of itchy eyes or foreign body sensation, to dentists complaining of cavities, and to specialists in ears, nose, and throat for dry mouth and difficulty swallowing. Whenever possible, these complaints should be documented as outlined by the Scripps criteria listed above. When the syndrome is limited to dry mouth and dry eyes, symptomatic treatment to prevent corneal damage and loss of teeth should be the aim of therapy. The use of artificial tears every 3-6 hours, and saliva substitutes, as well as fastidious oral hygiene and avoidance of sugary food and drink products is important. Any medications or lifestyle choices (e.g., smoking) that may be producing or worsening the condition should be modified or eliminated as much as possible.

A diagnosis of primary Sjögren's syndrome calls for a similar supportive approach, but when associated with extraglandular involvement, additional therapy with corticosteroids and cytotoxic drugs may be necessary. Bromhexine, a secretagogue, has been used in Europe, but there are no conclusive double-blind studies of its efficacy. Supplementation with essential fatty acids and vitamins have been studied without definite evidence of efficacy but many subjective reports of improvement.

When SS is present in association with a connective tissue disease like SLE, RA, PSS, etc., or secondary to some other condition like lymphoma, in addition to symptomatic treatment, further treatment is dictated by the primary condition. Patients with extra-glandular or systemic involvement may require steroid and/or immunosuppressive therapy.

SUGGESTED READINGS

1. Marx RE, Hartman KS, Rethman KV. A prospective study comparing incisional labial to incisional parotid biopsies in the detection and confirmation of sarcoidosis, Sjögren's disease, sialosis and lymphoma. J. Rheumatol. 1988; 15:21-9.

2. Fox RI, Howell FV, Bane RC, Michelson P. Primary Sjögren's syndrome: Clinical and immunopathologic features. Sem Arthritis Rheum. 1984; 14:77-105.

3. Fox RI, Robinson CA, Curd JC, Kozin F, Howell FV. Sjögren's syndrome—proposed criteria for classification. Arthritis Rheum. 1986; 29:577-85.

Chapter 32

Fibromyalgia (Fibrositis)

Primary figromyalgia is a common disorder that occurs most frequently in middle-aged women. The primary symptoms are aches, pain and stiffness in muscles, at periarticular and articular sites, tendon insertions, and over bony prominences. Often accompanying the pain are systemic complaints such as insomnia and lack of restorative sleep, fatigue, tension headaches, and irritable bowel syndrome. When these symptoms develop in patients with some other underlying illness, it is called secondary fibromyalgia. It is therefore necessary to exclude underlying conditions such as polymyalgia rheumatica, systemic lupus erythematosus, rheumatoid arthritis, endocrine causes like hypothyroidism, acromegaly, hyperparathyroidism, and polymyositis or metabolic myopathies before making the diagnosis. Widespread osteoarthritis and bursitis or tendonitis must also be excluded, and underlying depression with secondary fibromyalgia should also be identified when present, since treatment will require much larger doses of tricyclic antidepressants than those used in primary fibromyalgia.

DIAGNOSTIC CRITERIA

Some physicians are skeptical that fibromyalgia truly is a "disease" because of the lack of definitive histopathology. However, patients with this syndrome provide a very distinct and consistent history and physical examination findings. Several criteria for diagnosis have been proposed. We favor those proposed by Yunus et al. in 1981.

I. Obligatory Criteria:
   1. generalized aches and pains or prominent stiffness involving 3 or more anatomic sites for at least three months.
   2. absence of secondary causes.

II. Major Criteria:
  1. Presence of at least five typical and consistent tender points.

III. Minor Criteria:
  1. Modulation of symptoms by physical activity (worse with too much or too little exercise)
  2. Modulation of symptoms by weather (better in warm, dry weather and worse in cold or humid weather)
  3. Aggravation by anxiety or stress
  4. Poor sleep
  5. General fatigue or tiredness
  6. Anxiety
  7. Chronic headache
  8. Irritable bowel syndrome
  9. Subjective swelling.
  10. Numbness

These criteria were 96% sensitive and 100% specific in their population of 50 patients with primary fibromyalgia and 50 control volunteers matched for age, sex, and race.

TENDER POINTS

Yunus and his colleagues identified as many as 38 tender points in some patients. These are listed below in order of frequency of involvement in their population.

the upper border of the trapezius
medial part of the knees
lateral elbow
posterior iliac crest
lumbar spine area
medial elbow
sternomastoid muscles
dorsal spine area
costochondral junctions
bicipital tendon
sacroiliac area
cervical spine
medial scapular border
greater trochanter of the hip
suboccipital muscle insertion area.

Studies using a dolorimeter to quantitate applied pressure have demonstrated that fibromyalgia patients develop pain in tender points with much less pressure than controls. However, non-tender point areas have the same pain threshold in these patients as in controls. Another characteristic finding is diurnal variation in symptoms—much worse in the early morning and late evening.

A recent report identified 19 sites of anatomic tenderness as better discriminators between PFM patients and controls. Some of these sites overlap with those described earlier and cluster around the anterior shoulder and chest, the posterior scapula, and the medial knee.

Migraine headaches, irritable bowel syndrome, and a previous diagnosis of mitral valve prolapse are commonly reported by these patients.

ETIOLOGY AND PATHOPHYSIOLOGY

The etiology of this syndrome is not well understood. The term "fibrositis" is a misnomer because there is no histologic evidence of inflammation in either the muscle or fascia. One theoretical explanation for the patients' symptoms is the lack of restorative sleep. Patients complain of waking up tired and with aching, stiff muscles. They do not wake up rested. Studies of some patients with this disorder have demonstrated abnormal EEG patterns consisting of decreased amounts of stage 4 (deep, restorative) sleep. In further support of this theory, one study showed that the symptoms of muscle soreness and aching could be induced in a group of normal, healthy volunteers if their stage 4 sleep was repeatedly disturbed by a buzzer during three consecutive nights.

Elevated levels of CD4/CD8 ratio of lymphocytes, IL-1, and interferon alpha have recently been reported in some patients with fibromyalgia, suggesting an altered immune response as possibly another mechanism causing symptoms. Further, it has been recognized that the use of IL-2 and interferon alpha in oncology patients commonly produces symptoms of primary fibromyalgia syndrome. One study reports abnormally low high-energy phosphate levels in the painful muscles of patients with primary fibromyalgia. Recently, a possible association between the chronic fatigue syndrome and PFM has been proposed, and while they may likely be identical in some patients, others probably represent distinctly different syndromes.

TREATMENT

Treatment of patients with fibromyalgia must be comprehensive to maintain patient confidence. Most of these patients have already seen many other physicians who have either ignored their symptoms, failed to recognize the disorder, or provided inadequate therapy. As a result of this response to their symptoms, these patients are often angry or depressed by the time they come to see you.

Since insomnia and lack of restorative sleep may be the basis of the muscle pain symptoms, treatment should start by attempting to relieve the insomnia. Often very low doses of amitriptyline (10-25 mg) at night are enough to restore a normal deep sleep pattern and, in some patients, relieve significant pain. If amitriptyline is not well tolerated, other tricyclic drugs, such as doxepin, can be used. Imipramine, though a tricyclic anti-depressant, was not useful in these patients. Newer anti-depressant drugs, such as trazodone (Desyrel) 50 mg. q.h.s., and muscle relaxants, such as cyclobenzaprine (Flexeril) 10-30 mg q.h.s., may also be of benefit. In patients who do not tolerate or improve with any one of these drugs, low-dose oral thorazine (25-50 mg q.h.s.) can be quite helpful. The risk from long-term daily use of these agents is probably low but unknown. Patients should be encouraged to try to go off medication as soon as they feel better to keep their exposure to these drugs to the smallest effective dose.

In addition to improving sleep, adequate analgesia must be provided. In most cases, nonsteroidal anti-inflammatory drugs alone are inadequate to relieve aching and discomfort. However, used in combination with amitriptyline, synergistic effects are observed. Narcotics and steroids play *no role* in the treatment of this disorder. In fact, a response to steroids virtually excludes fibromyalgia as the diagnosis.

While the physician tries to restore or improve sleep and provide analgesia, the third part of the treatment plan can be instituted, consisting of active patient participation in the healing process. Aerobic exercise has been shown to be beneficial in relieving muscle discomfort although initially it may exacerbate the regional aches and pains. The exercise program should start with brisk walking and gradually build up to intensive aerobic exercises if tolerated by the patient. Since many patients with fibromyalgia tend to be sedentary and have poor muscle tone, getting them involved initially with an exercise program may be difficult. It is, however, an essential part of the therapeutic plan. Therapeutic massage and hot showers have also been reported to help.

A higher percentage of psychologic disturbances in patients with PFM than RA patients have been reported in some series, while others have found no difference, depending on the population studied and the diagnostic tools and criteria used. One study in the psychiatric literature suggests a higher prevalence of affective disorders among relatives of patients with PFM than RA patients, but this area is far from settled.

We must emphasize that PFM is a different syndrome from psychogenic rheumatism. These patients are tender all over as opposed to PFM patients who are tender only in discrete predictable sites. Psychogenic rheumatism patients do not experience relief with any treatment modality and deny diurnal variation in their symptoms since they hurt "all the time." While the course of PFM may be life-long with periods of marked relief, patients with psychogenic rheumatism rarely (if ever) improve.

SUGGESTED READINGS

1. Yunus M, Masi AT, Calabro JJ, Miller KA, Feigenbaum SL. Primary fibromyalgia (fibrositis): Clinical study of 50 patients with matched normal controls. Arthritis Rheum. 1981; 11:151-171.

2. Simms RW, Goldenberg DL, Felson DT, Mason JH. Tenderness in 75 anatomic sites—distinguishing fibromyalgia patients from controls. Arthritis Rheum. 1988; 31:182-7.

3. Bennett RM, Goldenberg DL, editors. The fibromyalgia syndrome. Rheum Dis Clin North Am. 1989; 15:1-191.

Chapter 33

Gout

Gout is a form of inflammatory arthritis associated with the presence of monosodium urate (MSU) crystals in synovial fluid. Symptoms are intermittent, severe, and involve only one or several joints early in the disease course. After years, the disease can become chronic and destructive and can involve many joints. Gout is chiefly a disease of middle-aged or older men and of postmenopausal women. Often there is a family history of gout. Both gout and asymptomatic hyperuricemia are frequently associated with other disorders such as obesity, hypertension, and hyperlipidemia.

Hyperuricemia (serum uric acid above 8 mg/dl by auto-analyzer) is a biochemical abnormality that is found in the majority of patients with gout (but *not* all). It is common in the general population (5%) and very common (18%) in hospitalized patients. However, only one in 40 hyperuricemic patients will develop symptoms related to uric acid excess (arthritis or renal stones).

CLINICAL MANIFESTATIONS

1. *Acute Gout*: Early attacks of gout are typically monoarticular or oligoarticular (4 or fewer joints) and affect lower extremity joints 95% of the time. The great toe, ankle, or knee will develop the sudden onset of moderate to severe pain with the typical acute attack lasting five to seven days. Less commonly, "petite" attacks present as milder pain lasting only hours or several days.
2. *Recurrent Gouty Arthritis*: Five to 10% of patients with acute gout will never have a recurrence of their symptoms—even if they are untreated. Most gouty patients will develop recurrent acute episodes within an average symptom-free interval of 11 months (range 3-36

months). As the number of recurrences increases, the interval between episodes shortens and the duration of each attack lengthens.

3. *Chronic Tophaceous Gout*: After several years to a decade or more of intermittent gout, the arthritis can become chronic (no symptom-free intervals) and polyarticular. This phase is marked by the presence of *tophi*, (urate crystal aggregates) in tendons, bursae, and subcutaneous tissues. In general, the higher the serum urate, the earlier the appearance and the more extensive the development of tophi.

PATHOGENESIS OF GOUT AND HYPERURICEMIA

Gout is the consequence of prolonged hyperuricemia and is mediated by various physical and inflammatory factors. Hyperuricemia is classified as *secondary* when associated with a disease, drug, or physiologic process known to elevate uric acid levels. It is considered *primary* if such an association cannot be made. Both primary and secondary hyperuricemia may be caused by (a) overproduction of uric acid or (b) renal underexcretion of uric acid.

1. *Primary Hyperuricemia*
   a. Increased production of uric acid (rare)
      HPRT deficiency
      PRPP synthetase overactivity
   b. Decreased renal excretion of uric acid (common)
   c. Idiopathic
2. Secondary Hyperuricemia
   a. Increased production of uric acid
      i. Increased nucleic acid turnover
         Myeloproliferative disorders
         Lymphoproliferative disorders
         Psoriasis
      ii. Increased catabolism of nucleotides
         Exercise
         Rhabdomyolysis
   b. Decreased renal excretion of uric acid
      i. Reduced renal functional mass
         Chronic renal failure
      ii. Decreased fractional excretion of uric acid
         Lead nephropathy (saturnine gout)

iii. Competitive excretion of organic acids
Ethanol ingestion
Starvation ketosis
Diabetic ketoacidosis
Salicylates (in low dose)
Ethambutol
Phenylbutazone
Diuretics (especially thiazides)

DIAGNOSIS

The *definitive* diagnosis of acute gouty arthritis is made by examining either synovial fluid or tophaceous deposits for the characteristic needle-like MSU crystals which show strong negative birefringence by compensated polarized light microscopy. The common practice of relying on the less specific findings of the classic gouty triad—acute monarthritis + hyperuricemia + symptomatic improvement on colchicine—may lead to mistaken diagnoses and poor treatment results. The differential diagnosis of acute monoarticular gout includes:

—septic arthritis (especially secondary to N. gonorrhoea)
—other crystal-induced arthropathies (pseudo-gout)
—palindromic rheumatism and rheumatoid arthritis
—traumatic arthritis
—sarcoid arthritis

Radiographic findings are usually minimal and non-diagnostic in the early phase of gout. After multiple acute episodes and certainly by the stage of chronic tophaceous gout, characteristic x-ray changes may occur. These include overhanging margins of bone and punched-out lesions.

TREATMENT OF GOUT

Management strategies for gout need to be individualized for the severity and frequency of the patient's symptoms as well as for the stage of disease, as categorized in Table 33.1.

The drugs used to treat gouty arthritis fall into two major classes: (1) those that reduce pain and swelling (anti-inflammatory agents) and (2) those that decrease serum urate levels (anti-hyperuricemic agents).

Table 33.1
Management strategies

Disease Stage	Acute Anti-inflamm. Therapy (see Table 2)	Maintenance Anti-inflamm. Therapy (see Table 3)	Anti-Hyperuricemic Therapy (see Table 4)
Asymptomatic Hyperuricemia	0	0	0*
Acute Mono-Articular	+	0	0
Recurrent Acute Arthritis	+	+	±
Chronic Tophaceous Gout	+	+	+

*Serum urate 12 mg/dl or greater should be evaluated. Levels in this range are often secondary to drugs or other underlying conditions (such as renal insufficiency), and these factors should be looked for.

Anti-inflammatory drugs currently available in this country have no beneficial effects on serum urate levels. Anti-hyperuricemic drugs, on the other hand, have no beneficial effect on the pain and swelling of acute gouty symptoms. Dramatic changes in serum urate caused by these drugs may in fact initiate or exacerbate gout.

ALLOPURINOL THERAPY

Allopurinol (Zyloprim or Lopurin) is widely used and highly effective means of reducing serum uric acid levels. Caution should be exercised in its use, especially in the following situations.

1. Any degree of *renal failure* (minimal to severe), especially if the patient is on *thiazide* diuretics. Initial allopurinol doses should be reduced according to the creatinine clearance (see Reference 4). Concomitant administration of cytotoxics is quite dangerous because of decreased clearance of these agents. Dose of the cytotoxic must be decreased accordingly.

Table 33.2
Pharmacologic Management of Acute Gouty Arthritis

Drug	Route	Dose	Major Adverse Effects	Relative Contraindictations
Colchicine	Oral	0.6 mg/hr (up to 12 doses)	Nausea and diarrhea acutely. Bone marrow suppression from overdose, as well as acute myopathy	Active peptic ulcer disease, liver disease, sepsis, bone marrow suppression
	IV	2 mg initially then 0.5 mg q 6-8 hr x 2 doses (Reduce for renal insufficiency)	Same as above	In addition to above, poor veins and recent therapy with large oral doses of colchicine
Indomethacin	Oral	150 mg initially, followed by 50 mg t.i.d.*	See Chapter 44.	Active or recurrent peptide ulcer disease, psychosis, dementia, cardiac or renal failure
Naproxen	Oral	1000 mg followed by 500 mg b.i.d.*	See Chapter 44.	Similar to indomethacin
Sulindac	Oral	400 mg followed by 200 mg t.i.d.*	See Chapter 44.	Similar to indomethacin
Ibuprofen	Oral	1200 mg followed by 800 mg t.i.d.*	See Chapter 44.	Similar to indomethacin
Corticosteroids	Intra-articular	10-40 mg	See Chapter 46.	Septic arthritis, bacterial cellulitis over the involved joints
ACTH	IM or subcut.	40-80 units	Sodium retention, muscle weakness, embryocidal	Pregnant or nursing mothers, CHF

*These dosees should only be given until symptoms abate. For maintenance doses see Table 33.3.

Table 33.3
Maintenance Anti-Inflammatory Therapy

Drug	Route	Dose	Major Adverse Effects
Colchicine	Oral	0.6 mg q.d. to t.i.d.	Nausea, diarrhea, peripheral neuropathy
Indomethacin	Oral	25-50 mg t.i.d.	Gastric irritation, headaches, fluid retention
Naproxen	Oral	375-500 mg b.i.d.	Gastric irritation
Sulindac	Oral	200 mg b.i.d.	Gastric irritation
Ibuprofen	Oral	600-800 mg t.i.d.	Gastric irritation

Table 33.4
Anti-hyperuricemic Agents*

Drug	Route	Dose	Major Adverse Effects	Relative Contraindications
Probenecid	Oral	Start with 250 mg t.i.d. and increase every 1-2 weeks to 1 gm t.i.d.	Gastric irritation	Overproduction of uric acid, uric acid stones, GFR below 50% of normal, concurrent salicylate administration
Sulfinpyrazone	Oral	Start with 100 mg b.i.d. and increase every 1-2 weeks up to 400 mg b.i.d.	Gastric irritation	Same as above.
Allopurinol	Oral	Initial: 100-150 mg q.d. up to 300-800 mg q.d. In renal failure, dose *must* be adjusted	Gastric irritation skin rash, vasculitis, granulomatous hepatitis	Liver disease, bone marrow suppression, administration of cytotoxic agents

*The goal of hypouricemic therapy is to reduce serum urate to between 5 and 6 mg/dl.

2. *Active gouty symptoms*. Any of the uric acid-lowering agents (Table 33.4) may precipitate or exacerbate gout if they are initiated without anti-inflammatory coverage.

Initial therapy should start at 100 mg per day with serum uric acid levels monitored frequently. The dose can be slowly increased until the uric acid level is 5-6 mg/dl. This approach will avoid the severe life-threatening complications of allopurinol, which include a dose-dependent bone marrow suppression and an idiosyncratic hypersensitivity reaction associated with liver and kidney failure and a 20% risk of death.

COLCHICINE

Colchicine has been used as an oral antigout medication for centuries. Until the advent of NSAIDs, it was the only consistently successful form of therapy for acute gout and a rapid clinical response to colchicine was considered diagnostic of gout. Although colchicine is still frequently used as a maintenance agent to prevent gouty recurrences, its role in treating *acute gout* has been widely supplanted by the NSAIDs. This is due to the frequent gastrointestinal symptoms resulting from high-dose oral colchicine use. It is also now recognized that the therapeutic actions of colchicine are not specific for gout. The other two common forms of crystalline arthropathy (calcium pyrophosphate dihydrate and hydroxyapatite) respond to colchicine as do other conditions like sarcoid arthritis, erythema nodosum, serum sickness, and Familial Mediterranean Fever. The response of these latter conditions to colchicine is usually far less dramatic than that observed in acute gout.

A. Use of colchicine in acute gout

1. *Oral Administration*

   The effectiveness of any agent in treating acute gout depends on how soon it is started after the initial symptoms occur. In the case of colchicine, if symptoms have existed for more than 12 hours, the likelihood of a prompt therapeutic response drops off. For this reason and because of frequent GI side effects, oral colchicine is *not* the treatment of choice when therapy cannot be initiated promptly. However, patients that are able to recognize the very earliest symptoms of acute gout and initiate treatment immediately can frequently abort the painful episode. This type of rapid response is still considered by many to be "diagnostic" of gout.

The two most popular *oral* dosing schedules for colchicine are

a. One tablet (0.6 mg) is taken at hourly intervals until:
   —symptoms subside,
   —cramping abdominal pain, diarrhea, nausea, and vomiting occur,
   —or a maximum of 12 hourly doses (7 mg) has been given in 24 hours

   After the first day, the dose should be decreased to one tablet b.i.d. or t.i.d.

b. Two tablets (1.2 mg) taken immediately and then one tablet every two hours, therefore, a maximum of 12 tablets in the first day and a maintenance dose of 0.6 mg. b.i.d. or t.i.d. thereafter. This program has fewer GI problems, but relief of symptoms is no more rapid than with less toxic NSAIDs.

Other toxicities from oral colchicine in acute gout are unusual; however, patients who are septic, neutropenic, or on other forms of bone marrow suppressants *should not* be given colchicine by any route.

2. *Intravenous Administration* (avoid giving it except under supervision)

   I.V. colchicine should be restricted to hospitalized patients. It is given as 2 mg (4 ml) of injectable colchicine diluted in 20 ml saline and administered through a large peripheral vein over 20 minutes. Colchicine that extravasates outside the vein is very irritating and may cause tissue damage. If prompt response is not seen in the several hours following intravenous colchicine, repeat I.V. doses of 1 mg may be given at six hour intervals to a maximum of *4 mg* during the ENTIRE episode. If there has been no relief, consider alternative treatment.

   An anticipated consequence of this form of therapy is marrow suppression and neutropenia. In very ill, infected or marrow-suppressed patients, this form of gout therapy is contraindicated, as mentioned earlier. Deaths have been seen.

B. Maintenance Use of Colchicine

Between acute episodes of gout, oral colchicine may be used to reduce the frequency and severity of "gouty flares." The usual maintenance dose is 1 to 3 tablets daily in divided doses. Most patients develop GI symptoms on this schedule, however, so b.i.d. is more commonly prescribed.

This form of therapy is considered quite safe with side effects being rare. Chronic colchicine use may lead to *colchicine myopathy and neuropathy,* which is frequently unrecognized or misdiagnosed. These conditions occur primarily in patients with *chronic renal failure* and may appear even after the patient has been on colchicine for 10 or 20 years. Serum creatine kinase levels become elevated, an axonal polyneuropathy is confirmed on nerve conduction studies, and a proximal myopathy is seen clinically and on EMG. The symptoms slowly abate after stopping colchicine.

SUGGESTED READINGS

1. Boss GR, Seegmiller JE. Hyperuricemia and gout: Classification, complications and management. N Engl J Med. 1979; 300:1459-68.

2. Fox IH, Kelley WN. Management of gout. JAMA. 1979; 242:361-64.

3. Liang MH, Fries JF. Asymptomatic hyperuricemia: The case for conservative management. Ann Intern Med. 1978; 88:666-70.

4. Hande KR, Noone RM, Stone WJ. Severe allopurinol toxicity. Description and guidelines for prevention in patients with renal insufficiency. Am J Med. 1984; 76:47-56

5. Kund RW, Duncan G, Watson D, et al. Colchicine myopathy and neuropathy. N Engl J Med. 1987; 316:1562-68.

Chapter 34

Other Crystal-Induced Arthropathies

I. Calcium Pyrophosphate Dihydrate (CPPD) Deposition)

A. *Definition*

CPPD deposition is a disease characterized by calcification of articular and meniscal cartilage (chondrocalcinosis) and a crystalline synovitis analogous to that induced by monosodium urate in gout. CPPD deposits are found only in joints and neighboring tendons. Soft tissue calcium deposits in arteries, skin, brain, heart valves, or muscles are the more common calcium hydroxyapatite (basic calcium) salt. CPPD deposits are present in 5% of cadaver knees with the percentage increasing markedly in the elderly.

B. *Clinical Manifestations*

CPPD deposition disease is a "great imitator" because it can mimic most types of arthritis. These various clinical patterns of CPPD disease have been classified by the arthropathy they resemble.

Pseudogout—Type A
Pseudorheumatoid Arthritis—Type B
Pseudo-osteoarthritis (inflammatory)—Type C
Pseudo-osteoarthritis (non-inflammatory)—Type D
Asymptomatic CPPD Deposition—Type E
Pseudoneuropathic joint—Type F
Occasionally CPPD may also resemble ankylosing spondylitis or rheumatic fever.

In non-familial disease, the onset of symptoms occurs at a mean age of 57 (range 38-92). Symptoms may be quite mild with little more than transient aching or may be severe with marked swelling and fever. The duration of attacks varies from a few hours to several weeks. The average attack is longer than that in gout. Some patients never have circumscribed attacks, but rather present with chronic swelling of wrists and MCP joints, mimicking rheumatoid arthritis. The knee is the most commonly involved joint, followed by the wrist, ankle, elbow, hip, and shoulder. The sacroiliac joint or spine may occasionally be involved. In contrast to gout, the MTP joints are rarely involved.

C. *Disease Associations*

As with gout, CPPD disease may be idiopathic or familial or occur in association with other diseases, such as:

1. General associations
   - aging
   - renal failure
2. Other joint diseases
   - osteoarthritis
   - ochronosis
3. Metabolic disorders
   - hypothyroidism
   - hyperparathyroidism
   - hemochromatosis
   - hypophosphatasia
   - hypomagnesemia
   - Wilson's disease

D. *Diagnosis and Laboratory Findings*

The characteristic feature of active CPPD disease is the demonstration of CPPD crystals in synovial fluid by compensated polarized microscopy. The crystals are usually intracellular and may appear as narrow needles (monoclinic form) resembling gout or broad rhomboid crystals (triclinic form). CPPD crystals show a *weakly positive birefringence,* contrasting with the strong negative birefringence of gout crystals. The synovial fluid WBC count is usually above 15,000/mm with 95% being PMNs. In chronic or subsiding effusions, the cell count may be much lower.

Chondrocalcinosis is observed on radiographs in the vast majority of patients with CPPD disease. The knee is the most frequent site with calcification in both meniscal and hyaline cartilage. Other frequently involved joints are the symphysis pubis, shoulder, hip, and triangular cartilage of the wrist. Other x-ray changes include loss of cartilage space and juxta-articular bone cysts. During acute attacks, crystals are "shed" from the cartilage, and the x-ray appearance of chondrocalcinosis may diminish or disappear.

The sedimentation rate (ESR) may be moderately elevated in acute attacks. A work-up for an underlying metabolic disease or other predisposing factor is recommended in symptomatic patients under the age of 65. The work-up includes: serum calcium, phosphorus and magnesium, T_4 and TSH, serum iron and iron-binding capacity, alkaline phosphatase, creatinine, and BUN.

E. *Management*

Indomethacin and other NSAIDs are effective in controlling the inflammation of CPPD-induced synovitis. In refractory cases, colchicine may be useful as an additive agent. In cases where NSAIDs are not tolerated, colchicine alone or with intra-articular corticosteroids may be beneficial.

II. Calcium Hydroxyapatite (Basic Calcium) Crystal Disease

A. *Definition*

Hydroxyapatite crystal disease may present as an acute periarthritis (tendonitis or bursitis) or as an acute or subacute arthropathy. Like CPPD disease, hydroxyapatite deposition is a frequent finding in severe osteoarthritis. Other clinical settings in which hydroxyapatite crystals are observed include chronic renal dialysis patients and an arthropathy in elderly females (mean age 75) with unilateral or bilateral rotator cuff lysis and severe, destructive, glenohumeral arthritis (termed "apatite-associated destructive arthropathy" or "Milwaukee shoulder"). This latter condition can also occur in the knee.

B. *Laboratory Studies*

The synovial fluid ranges from minimally inflammatory to markedly inflammatory. The cells may be either PMNs or monocytes. The calcium hydroxyapatite crystals are *not* easily observed by standard or compensated, polarized microscopy. Aggregates of these tiny crystals may appear as "shiny silver coins" on wet mount of synovial fluids. Most commonly, the crystal aggregates are detected on freshly obtain synovial fluid using a calcium stain (alizarin red or von Kossa).

C. *Management*

The optimal medical management of acute and chronic hydroxyapatite symptoms is with either NSAIDs or colchicine and is similar to that of CPPD disease.

SUGGESTED READINGS

1. McCarty DJ. Calcium pyrophosphate dihydrate crystal deposition disease: Nomenclature and diagnostic criteria. Ann Intern Med. 1977; 87:240-2

2. Dieppe PA, Alexander GJM, Jones HE, et al. Pyrophosphate arthropathy: A clinical and radiological study of 105 cases. Ann Rheum Dis. 1982; 41:371-6.

3. Dieppe PA, Doherty M, MacFarlane GD, et al. Apatite associated destructive arthritis. Br J Rheumatol. 1984; 23:84-91.

4. Paul H, Reginato AJ, Schumacher HR. Alizarin red staining as a screening test to detect calcium compounds in synovial fluid. Arthritis Rheum. 1983; 26:1910-200.

5. McCarty DJ, ed. Crystalline disposition diseases. Rheum Dis Clin NA 1988; 14:253-495.

Chapter 35

Seronegative Spondyloarthropathies

ANKYLOSING SPONDYLITIS, REITER'S SYNDROME, PSORIATIC ARTHRITIS AND INFLAMMATORY BOWEL DISEASE-ASSOCIATED ARTHRITIS

The seronegative spondyloarthropathies constitute a group of arthritic disorders linked by shared features, including clinical manifestations, radiologic findings, and a strong association with the histocompatibility antigen HLA-B27. The clinical features that characterize the spondyloarthropathies are:

—involvement of sacroiliac joints and spine,
—peripheral arthritis (primarily lower extremities),
—inflammation of entheses (where tendons attach to bone),
—extra-articular features (mucocutaneous and gastrointestinal),
—onset usually under the age of 40,
—males more symptomatic than females,
—familial clustering, and
—absence of rheumatoid factor.

The diseases calcified as seronegative spondyloarthropathies are:

Ankylosing spondylitis
Reiter's syndrome with or without spondylitis
Psoriatic arthritis with or without spondylitis
Inflammatory bowel disease-associated arthritis
Reactive arthritis (*Yersinia, Salmonella, Shigella*)
Juvenile ankylosing spondylitis

Ankylosing Spondylitis (AS)

A. *Clinical Manifestations*:
The insidious onset (over weeks to months) of low back, buttock or thigh pain is the most common early symptom. The pain and stiffness are typically worse in the morning or after immobility and improve with activity. This pattern distinguishes the inflammatory spondyloarthropathies from other common causes of low back pain. Except for hips and shoulders, peripheral arthritis is usually transient. Women and children have more peripheral involvement and generally milder symptoms overall. In males, progressive involvement of the lumbar, thoracic, and cervical spine results in increased pain, decreased flexibility, and restricted respiratory excursion. When posture maintenance and flexibility have *not* been emphasized as a critical component of therapy, thoracolumbar kyphosis, anterior flexion of the cervical spine, and flexion contractures of the hip lead to the classic "hunched over" appearance of ankylosing spondylitis.

Extra-articular manifestations include iritis (20-40%) and aortitis (5%). The aortitis may lead to conduction abnormalities and aortic valve insufficiency. Upper lobe fibrosis suggestive of tuberculosis may develop in patients with severe disease.

B. *Laboratory Findings*:
Rheumatoid factor is absent, and the sedimentation rate is often moderately elevated. Radiographic evidence of sacroiliac involvement is present within the first several months of symptoms. Plain radiographs of the sacroiliac joints show blurring, erosions, marginal sclerosis, and, eventually fusion. Bone scans and CT can be useful in establishing early sacroiliac involvement. Lumbar straightening, erosive remodeling (squaring) of involved vertebrae, and syndesmophyte formation are present in established disease. HLA-B27 antigen is present in 95% of white patients with AS, in 50% of black patients, and in 6-8% of normal individuals. This test is not useful as a routine screening test.

C. *Treatment*
Postural deformity can be minimized with good physical therapy supervision including:

—stretching and strengthening exercises
—swimming and stationary bicycling

—attention to correct posture throughout the day
—firm mattress, sleeping on side.

Anticipated reduced chest wall expansion makes cessation of smoking mandatory. Family education and genetic counseling (10-20% of offspring may develop AS) are important. Eventual ankylosis of the costovertebral joints leads to impaired chest expansion and the risk of pneumonia. Since most respiratory motion in these patients depends on the diaphragm, spinal anesthesia should be avoided. Intubation during anesthesia also requires expert care to avoid hyperextension of the neck with possible cervical spine fracture.

NSAIDs are useful with indomethacin considered by many to be the drug of choice. Sulfasalazine (2 gm p.o. q.d.) may also be helpful. Narcotics should be avoided.

Reiter's Syndrome and Other Reactive Arthritides

A. *Clinical Manifestations*:
Classic Reiter's syndrome presents as the clinical triad of urethritis, arthritis, and conjunctivitis, usually following a genitourinary infection with either *Chlamydia* or *Ureaplasma*. The complete triad is not necessary to make the diagnosis of RS. Other common features include oral ulcers, balanitis, uveitis, and keratoderma. Low back pain (sacroiliitis) and foot and ankle symptoms are the most common joint complaints. The syndrome may remit after a single episode or may become chronic (similar to AS). RS is considered a *"post-venereal reactive arthritis"* since the genitourinary infection leads to an inflammatory reaction in joints that are not felt to be directly infected with the organism. *Post-dysentery reactive arthritis* is similar to RS but is associated with enteric infections with *Yersinia, Salmonella, Shigella,* and *Campylobacter.*

B. *Laboratory Findings*:
HLA-B27 is present in 75-80% of RS patients. Its presence predicts those at risk for sacroiliitis and uveitis. Sacroiliac films show unilateral or asymmetrical inflammation. Other radiographic findings include diffuse periosteitis and asymmetric syndesmophytes.

C. *Treatment*
Physical therapy can improve symptoms and prevent deformities. NSAIDs are helpful during acute flares and for maintenance.

Tetracycline should be used to treat the urethritis. Intra-articular steroid injections for oligoarthritis and topical corticosteroids for cutaneous lesions are useful adjuncts. Lesions of the penis are treated with low dose (1%) hydrocortisone topically. Recalcitrant RS may occasionally require sulfasalazine (2–3 gm per day) or methotrexate (7.5 to 15 mg per *week*).

Psoriatic Arthritis (PsA)

A. Clinical Manifestations

Between 5 and 10% of patients with psoriasis will develop inflammatory arthritis. The onset of joint symptoms may coincide with development of skin disease or may precede or follow the skin manifestations by months or years. Several distinct types of PsA have been described.

Type I *Asymmetric oligo- or polyarthritis* occurs in 50% of patients with PsA and primarily involves the DIP and PIP joints of hands and feet presenting as "sausage digits." Other commonly involved joints are hips, knees, ankles, and wrists. Nail pitting and onycholysis are frequent associated findings.

Type II *Symmetric oligo- or polyarthritis* accounts for 25% of PsA and is more aggressive and destructive disease than Type I PsA. The joints involved and the characteristic nail changes are similar to Type I.

Type III Psoriatic spondyloarthritis represents 25% of PsA and most closely resembles Reiter's syndrome in both clinical and radiographic manifestations. Peripheral joint symptoms may follow spinal involvement.

Arthritis mutilans is a severe, relentless course of destructive arthritis that may be seen with any of the three types of PsA. *Inflammatory eye disease* (conjunctivitis or iridocyclitis) may complicate PsA and should be treated to prevent permanent visual impairment.

B. *Laboratory Findings*:

Patients with PsA are rheumatoid factor negative. HLA-B27 is positive in 50-60% of PsA patients with spondylitis. Radiographic changes include erosions of small joints, osteolysis of terminal phalanges, and subperiosteal bone apposition (periostitis). Sacroiliac changes in Type III are usually unilateral and syndesmophytes are asymmetric and nonmarginal.

C. *Treatment*:

The optimal treatment of PsA includes physical therapy, rest, orthotics and anti-inflammatory therapy. Aspirin or non-steroidal anti-inflammatory drugs (NSAIDs), along with occasional intra-articular steroid injections, are sufficient drug therapy for most cases of PsA. In more resistant cases, the following drugs have been used to treat PsA.

Hydroxychloroquine (Plaquenil) 200-400 mg per day. There may be a small risk of exacerbating the underlying psoriasis.

Intramuscular gold salts (regimen same as for rheumatoid arthritis)

Methotrexate (7.5 to 15 mg weekly—Chapter 45)

Oral corticosteroids—used only short-term

Inflammatory Bowel Disease (IBD)-Associated Spondylitis

Patients with ulcerative colitis and Crohn's disease may develop a peripheral arthritis that closely resembles rheumatoid arthritis except the patients are rheumatoid factor negative. This form of arthritis tends to wax and wane with the bowel disease. Patients with these forms of inflammatory bowel disease may also develop a spondylitis identical to ankylosing spondylitis. The spondylitis form of IBD-associated arthritis does not change with the bowel disease and is treated as one would ankylosing spondylitis. In both forms of IBD-associated arthritis, sulfasalazine (Azulfadine 1 gm po bid) may be used to treat both bowel and joint symptoms.

SUGGESTED READINGS

1. Carette S, Graham D, Little H, et al. The natural disease course of ankylosing spondylitis. Arthritis Rheum. 1983; 26:186-90.

2. Dougados M, Boumier P, Amor B. Sulphasalazine in ankylosing spondylitis: a double-blind controlled study in 60 patients. Brit Med J. 1986; 293-911-14.

3. Arnett FC. Seronegative spondyloarthropathies. Bull Rheum Dis. 1987; 37:1-12.

4. Moll JMH, Haslock I, Macrae IF, Wright V. Associations between ankylosing spondylitis, psoriatic arthritis, Reiter's disease, the intestinal arthropathies, and Beçhet's syndrome. Medicine. 1974; 53:343-64.

Chapter 36

Degenerative Joint Disease

Degenerative joint disease is also known as osteoarthritis (OA) or osteoarthrosis. It is primarily a degenerative disease of articular cartilage which is accompanied by an overgrowth of bone. It is the most common type of arthritis and usually becomes clinically apparent in people over the age of 40, although degenerative changes may begin in the third decade.

The overall frequency of osteoarthritis is equal in men and women, although under the age of 45, there are more men with osteoarthritis while over the age of 55, women predominate. There is no significant relationship between osteoarthritis and race, heredity, climate, or geographic location, with a few exceptions—for example, the decreased frequency of hip osteoarthritis noted in the Chinese population.

Cartilage and Osteoarthritis

Cartilage facilitates the smooth gliding of a joint as it moves through its range of motion. To a lesser extent, it also provides some load support. It is composed of chondrocytes, the cellular element, and an acellular or matrix component. The matrix is composed of three elements:

1. water, which accounts for over 70% of its content,
2. Type II collagen, which gives articular cartilage its structural framework and also modulates the amount of proteoglycan hydration, and
3. proteoglycans, which exist mainly in an aggregated form and are imbedded in the collagen mesh. They are extremely hydrophilic. Proteoglycans release water with compression of the cartilage and regain it following decompression, thus giving cartilage its resiliency. They consist of subunits composed of glycosaminoglycans (chondroitin-6-sulfate, chondroitin-4-sulfate, and keratan sulfate), covalently attached to a protein core. Proteoglycans are non-

covalently bound to hyaluronic acid by link proteins to form proteoglycan aggregates which anchor in the collagen mesh.

Osteoarthritic cartilage undergoes a number of changes proceeding from biochemical to morphologic changes. Early in the course of osteoarthritis, there is a decrease in proteoglycan aggregability, alterations in collagen, an early increase in water content, and increased enzymatic activity with proliferation of chondrocytes. As a result of these early biochemical changes, distinctive morphologic changes occur. Osteoarthritic cartilage is characterized by fissuring and focal loss of cartilage, subchondral microfractures, attempts at repair characterized by marginal formations of bone and cartilage (known as osteophytes), and subchondral sclerosis and eburnation.

Classification of Osteoarthritis

I. Primary
  A. Idiopathic
  B. Primary generalized osteoarthritis
  C. Erosive inflammatory osteoarthritis
II. Secondary
  A. Inflammatory
    Rheumatoid arthritis
    Axial arthropathies
    Septic arthritis
    Recurrent crystalline synovitis
  B. Biochemical
    Trauma—acute, chronic
    Neuropathic arthropathy
    Avascular necrosis
  C. Endocrine related
    Diabetes mellitus
    Acromegaly
    Sex hormone abnormalities
    Iatrogenic Cushing's syndrome
    Hypothyroidism
  D. Metabolic
    Chondrocalcinosis
    Gout
    Hemochromatosis

Ochronosis
Wilson's disease
Paget's disease

E. Developmental abnormalities
Congenital hip dysplasia
Slipped capital femoral epiphysis
Legg-Calvé-Perthes disease
Femoral head and neck abnormalities
Morquio's syndrome

Etiology

The etiology of osteoarthritis is unknown but appears to involve multiple factors which interplay to a variable extent and lead to a final common pathway consisting of cartilage loss and attempts at repair. Genetic, endocrine, metabolic, inflammatory, and biomechanical loading lead to eventual chondrocyte injury, collagen, disruption, and subchondral microfractures. Though all three events occur, it is unclear which is the initial event. As an end-result, there is a release of degradative enzymes from the chondrocytes, resulting in cartilage breakdown. There is a genetic predisposition, in some patients and with some joints, particularly for Heberden's nodes, which appears to be autosomal dominant in females and autosomal recessive in males.

The occupational risks of developing osteoarthritis are uncertain. For example there is a possible association with jobs involving repetitive trauma. However, pneumatic drill operators did not have an increased incidence of osteoarthritis of the wrists or elbows.

Other factors which play a role in osteoarthritis include joint instability such as occurs with hypermobility syndromes, and neuroarthropathy. Since osteoarthritis is a disease of the middle-aged and elderly, it is theorized that aging cartilage has a decreased ability to resist mechanical stress. However, not all elderly individuals develop osteoarthritis, and, until recently, no specific biochemical changes have been found in aging articular cartilage.

Hormonal factors also may play a role. There is an increased prevalence of osteoarthritis in post-menopausal women. Estrogen-treated mice are protected from osteoarthritis, while androgen-treated mice exhibit increased incidence. Other hormones also play a role. There is an increased frequency of osteoarthritis in patients with acromegaly, hypothyroidism, and diabetes.

The role of obesity is unclear, since while the best association is with osteoarthritis of the knees (weight-bearing joints), there is also an association with OA of the hands, suggesting a metabolic association rather than simple increased load on the joints. Secondary degenerative changes are also seen in the inflammatory arthritides such as gout and rheumatoid arthritis.

Clinical Characteristics

Symptoms include deep, aching joint pain that occurs with weight-bearing and/or activity and is relieved by rest. Because it is a local joint disorder, OA usually involves only a few joints and has no systemic manifestations. Morning stiffness may be present but is localized to the few joints involved and is brief, lasting no longer than 15 to 30 minutes. Signs associated with osteoarthritis include local joint tenderness, creaking, grating or cracking of the joint, and palpable osteophytes. Large joint effusions are usually not present. An important point to remember is that in the hands joint deformity occurs but function is preserved. It is not uncommon to have very "knobby-looking" hands but to maintain good function with very little pain. This is different from osteoarthritis of weight-bearing joints such as hips and knees in which functional loss occurs early and parallels radiographic changes.

In the hands, osteophytes are known as Heberden's nodes when present at distal interphalangeal joints and Bouchard's nodes when present at proximal interphalangeal joints. Characteristically, the MCP joints and the wrists are spared in primary osteoarthritis. The only area typically involved in the hands is the first metacarpal-carpal joint which may sublux. Other characteristic locations include the hips, the knees, and the cervical and lumbar spine. Although the ankle is a weight-bearing joint, it is not involved in primary osteoarthritis. The toes are also spared expect for the first metatarsophalangeal joint or bunion joint, which is often the first joint involved by the osteoarthritic process.

Laboratory Findings

Since osteoarthritis is a local joint disorder, it has no laboratory features of a systemic nature. Blood counts and chemistry profile are normal. Rheumatoid factor, ANA, and sedimentation rate are usually normal or negative. In the elderly population, these serologic tests may be abnormal in association with age alone. Synovial fluid findings in osteoarthritis show normal glucose and protein determinations and a synovial white blood cell count of less than 1,000/mm^3 with less than 25% polymorphonuclear leukocytes.

Radiographic Findings

Peripheral joints demonstrate joint space narrowing due to the loss of cartilage, subchondral bony sclerosis or eburnation, osteophytes, and subchondral cysts. In the spine, there may be disc degeneration with a decreased disc space and sclerosis as well as anterior, posterior, and/or apophyseal joint spurs. In the cervical and lumbar spine, oblique views are helpful to evaluate the neural foramina whenever a radicular component is present.

Clinical Patterns and Associations

A. *Primary generalized osteoarthritis* occurs primarily in middle-aged females and is characterized by osteoarthritis in multiple joints including the DIPs, the PIPs the first MCC joints, knees, first MTP, and lumbosacral and cervical spine. The inheritance pattern is similar to that of Heberden's nodes.

B. *Erosive inflammatory osteoarthritis* is characterized by episodes of painful inflammation of the DIP and PIP joints with erosive changes of these joints. Erosive changes elsewhere should lead one to suspect other diagnostic possibilities. This variant of osteoarthritis is characterized serologically by a negative rheumatoid factor and a normal or only slightly elevated sedimentation rate.

C. *Chondromalacia patellae.* Since the availability of arthroscopy, a more correct term to denote the symptom complex consisting of knee pain, particularly on climbing stairs, in association with a non-inflammatory effusion would be patellofemoral dysfunction. This condition occurs predominantly in young athletic individuals and is often associated with patellar crepitance and may be associated with a chronic laterally subluxing patella. Many patients may have symptoms of patellofemoral dysfunction but arthroscopically have no evidence of fragmentation or friability of the patella and thus do not have chondromalacia. This is important since it appears that patients with patellofemoral dysfunction are not at worse risk for the subsequent development of osteoarthritis.

D. *Diffuse idiopathic skeletal hyperostosis* (DISH), also known as ankylosing hyperostosis, appears predominantly in middle-aged men; 30% have associated diabetes mellitus, and 34% are HLA B-27 positive. Radiographically, it is characterized by five features: (1) flowing ligamentous ossification of four or more contiguous vertebrae, (2) normal disc height, (3) no apophyseal or sacroiliac involvement, (4) olecranon and calcaneal spurs, and (5) extra-spinal ligamentous calcification.

E. *Neuropathic arthropathy.* Diabetes mellitus is the most frequently associated condition. Diabetic neuropathy produces arthropathy of the midfoot; syphilitic tabes dorsalis leads to neuroarthropathy in the knees; and syringomyelia involves the joints of the upper extremity. Radiographically, it is characterized by exuberant osteophyte formation, often with extensive periarticular calcification and destruction and disorganization of normal joint anatomy.

F. *Calcium pyrophosphate dihydrate deposition disease* is commonly seen in association with osteoarthritis and should be considered as a possibility in a patient who looks like he has osteoarthritis but has symptomatic joints not commonly involved in primary osteoarthritis (see Chapter 34).

G. *Hydroxyapatite synovitis.* Hydroxyapatite (also known as basic calcium phosphate) crystals have been implicated in cases of mild synovitis occasionally seen in patients with osteoarthritis (see Chapter 34).

H. *Spinal stenosis.* Lumbar spinal stenosis is a condition in which the anteroposterior and lateral diameters of the bony spinal canal are narrower than normal and/or in which the shape of the canal in cross section is abnormal. The stenosis may be severe enough to cause compression of the nerve roots of the cauda equina in the lateral recess or in one or more of the neural foramina. This same condition can be seen in the cervical spine, and the patient may present with a cervical myelopathy. (See Chapters 14 and 16).

There are three types of stenosis: (1) developmental, in which the narrowing is usually uniform over almost the entire length of the lumbar bony canal, (2) degenerative stenosis which is usually segmental in nature. It is most marked opposite the intervertebral discs because of herniation opposite the posterior articular processes where the canal is compromised by osteophyte formation, and (3) combined lesions in which a congenitally narrowed spinal canal is further compromised by either disc herniation and/or osteophytosis.

Symptoms of lumbar stenosis include pain in the back or in one or both legs. The pain may be either constant or intermittent, and it frequently resembles claudication due to arterial occlusion; for example, it becomes worse with exercise and is relieved by rest. One key feature of lumbar spinal stenosis is that not only does the patient have to stop walking, but he or she often has to sit down in order to relieve the pain due to spinal stenosis. In contrast to arterial claudication, the patient can use an exercise bicycle without symptoms because the flexed posture relieves some of the stenosis. There may be diminution or altered sensation in the legs as well as variable weakness in the legs. Signs include spine movement limited by pain. There may be a patchy decrease in sensation to light touch and pinprick and variable decrease in strength. The diagnosis is made by a high index of suspicion and confirmed by CT of the spine with contrast or by MRI. In the cases of significant neurologic impairment, decompressive surgery is necessary.

Patients with cervical spinal stenosis with myelopathy may present primarily with a gait disturbance (see Chapter 14, Neck Pain).

Treatment

The major objectives in the treatment of osteoarthritis are the same as for all types of arthritis: (1) to relieve pain, (2) to minimize disability, and (3) to attempt to delay progression. Unfortunately, there is no current therapy in the treatment of osteoarthritis which has been able to delay progression of disease. There are some general considerations based on individual needs, including a proper balance of rest and exercise of the involved joints and correcting factors that produce excessive joint strain; for example, weight reduction is very useful in patients with hip and knee osteoarthritis. Good posture, a firm mattress, and altered patterns of lifting can be very beneficial in cervical and lumbar osteoarthritis. Physical therapy modalities such as hot packs, paraffin baths to the hands, massage, and range of motion exercises are also useful adjuncts, as are supportive devices such as cervical collars, splints, canes, and crutches, depending on the type and location of the osteoarthritis.

Analgesic and anti-inflammatory drugs form the backbone of drug therapy. Although osteoarthritis is the prototype of a degenerative non-inflammatory process, recent studies have shown a mild synovitis related to cartilage fragmentation and degradative enzymes present in the joint space.

Acetaminophen products are often used, but many rheumatologists prefer a medication that has both pain-relieving as well as anti-inflammatory potential. Aspirin has long been used as the initial drug since it is cheap and effective, unless contraindicated. The usual dosage for the treatment of osteoarthritis is between 6 and 10 tablets a day in divided doses. Unfortunately, side effects are common and occur at lower doses in the elderly. All of the non-steroidal anti-inflammatory agents (NSAIDs) currently on the market have been used successfully in the treatment of osteoarthritis. Indomethacin is touted as particularly beneficial in hip osteoarthritis although this may not be the case. Of recent interest is the observation that certain NSAIDs (aspirin, ibuprofen, fenoprofen) inhibit cartilage proteoglycan synthesis and theoretically may be deleterious in OA. However, years of experience with these drugs have not been associated with significant adverse effects and NSAIDS remain the cornerstone of drug therapy in OA. Analgesics such as Darvocet may be beneficial in cervical and lumbar osteoarthritis that is not responsive to NSAIDs, or in patients unable to tolerate anti-inflammatory drugs.

Narcotic analgesics should be reserved for use in patients with severe osteoarthritis that is not controlled by standard modalities including non-steroidal anti-inflammatory agents and physical therapy. Muscle relaxants also may play a role, particularly when muscle spasm is associated with cervical and lumbar osteoarthritis. Intra-articular steroids may occasionally be of benefit in a recalcitrant joint, once infection has been excluded. As a general rule, it is advised that there be no more than three injections in a single joint per year because of the concern of possible acceleration of the degenerative process. Debridement of joint mice through an arthroscope may be necessary in joints that "lock".

Total joint replacements have been of great value in patients with significant hip and/or knee osteoarthritis characterized by severe pain and/or significant disability that has not responded to a conservative regimen. Because the life of a prosthetic joint is limited to 10-15 years, surgery is preferentially recommended to patients over age 60. Results at good centers by well-trained orthopedic surgeons are very gratifying.

SUGGESTED READINGS

1. Moskowitz RW, Howell DW, Goldberg WM, Mankin HJ. *Osteoarthritis: Diagnosis and Management*. Philadelphia: WB Saunders, Co., 1984.

2. Lifschitz, ML, Harmon CE. Musculoskeletal problems in the elderly. In *Clinical Internal Medicine in the Aged*, RW Schrier (ed). Philadelphia: WB Saunders, 1982, pp 182-210.

Chapter 37

True Collagen Diseases

Considerable confusion surrounds the diseases associated with abnormalities of collagen and the other components of connective tissues. Part of the confusion dates back to 1942 when Klemperer and colleagues published a classic description of systemic lupus, scleroderma, dermatomyositis, and polyarteritis and used the term "collagen disease" to lump these entities together. The authors assumed the histologic changes of connective tissue homogenization and hyalinization found in each of these diseases were due to alterations of collagen. The use of the term "collagen disease" expanded to include many disorders characterized by multisystem involvement of organs rich in connective tissue. Over the past 40 years, detailed studies have failed to demonstrate any alteration of collagen structure or metabolism in most of these disorders. Gradually, the misnomer "collagen diseases" is being replaced by the more appropriate term "connective tissue diseases."

In contrast, several inherited disorders are characterized by true alterations in collagen structure and metabolism. These are the diseases rightfully called the true "collagen diseases."

Ehlers-Danlos Syndrome (EDS)

The Ehlers-Danlos syndrome is a spectrum of inherited disorders whose clinical manifestations range from mild to life-threatening. Several subsets of EDS have been described that are characterized by mode of inheritance, clinical features, and in some cases, specific biochemical defects.

In general, these patients tend to have hypermobile joints, frequent joint dislocations, and hyperextensible skin. In one subset, arterial wall rupture can occur with catastrophic results. Hemarthroses, scoliosis, and bowel rupture may also occur.

Marfan's Syndrome

Like Ehlers-Danlos syndrome, Marfan's syndrome encompasses several clinically distinct groups including classic (asthenic) form, nonasthenic form, Marfanoid hypermobility, congenital contractual arachnodactyly, and homocystinuric Marfanoid syndrome. The separate clinical phenotypes are presumed to be caused by distinct genetic defects, but all apparently share abnormal crosslinking of collagen. The clinical characteristics of Marfan's syndrome include skeletal, ocular, and cardiovascular problems.

Skeletal: The Marfanoid habitus is unusually tall with long thin extremities, muscular underdevelopment, and sparse subcutaceous fat.

Ocular: The most characteristic change is bilateral lens dislocation. Early onset cataracts and retinal detachments are also common.

Cardiovascular: Mitral valve prolapse and aneurysmal dilatation of the ascending aorta are common and may lead to acute catastrophic death in adulthood.

Patients with a marfanoid habitus and a family history of death at an early age should be evaluated by echocardiography to detect developing aneurysms of the thoracic aorta. Beta blockers appear to help delay this complication, and modifications in surgical treatment of the aneurysm have greatly improved prognosis for patients diagnosed early.

Homocystinuria

Homocystinuria is a rare metabolic disorder that shares many clinical features with Marfan's syndrome. It is an important diagnosis to consider since early therapy of some homocystinuric patients with pyridoxine or restricted diets may prevent the mental retardation and musculoskeletal abnormalities. They are also prone to early atherosclerosis.

Osteogenesis Imperfecta (OI)

Osteogenesis imperfecta is one of the more common inherited disorders of connective tissue. In three of the four types of OI (Types I, II and III) the molecular defect is in the synthesis of Type I collagen. The defect in Type IV OI is unknown. All four types of OI are characterized by brittle bones with multiple fractures, thin (blue) sclera, and dental abnormalities. The rationale for using calcium, fluoride, and vitamin D in these patients is very questionable.

SUGGESTED READINGS

1. Prockop DJ, Kivirikko KI, Tuderman L, Guzman NA. The biosynthesis of collagen and its disorders. (2 parts). N Engl J Med. 1979; 301:13-23, 77-84.

2. Prockop DJ, Kivirikko KI. Heritable diseases of collagen. N Engl J Med. 1984; 311:376-386.

3. Pyeritz RE, McKusick VA. The Marfan syndrome: Diagnosis and management. N Engl J Med. 1979; 300:772-777.

4. Gott VL, Pyeritz RE, Magovern GW Jr, Cameron DE, McKusick VA. Surgical treatment of aneurysms of the ascending aorta in the Marfan syndrome: Results of composite graft repair in 50 patients. N Engl J Med. 1986; 314:1070-1074.

Chapter 38

Metabolic Bone Diseases

The metabolic bone diseases comprise those syndromes characterized by abnormalities in the total amount or strength of the skeletal mass and its degree of mineralization. This chapter reviews the diagnosis and treatment of some of these disorders including osteoporosis, osteomalacia, and osteitis fibrosa. In addition, Paget's disease will also be discussed.

DEFINITION OF TERMS

Osteopenia: Reduction in bone density below normal levels. This is a radiologic finding that does not differentiate between osteoporosis and osteomalacia. By the time it is obvious radiographically, approximately 40-50% of the bone mass has been lost.

Osteoporosis: Is a clinical syndrome consisting of susceptibility to nontraumatic fractures of the vertebral bodies and fractures of the proximal femur and distal radius from minimal trauma in association with radiographic osteopenia. With the advent of more sensitive measures of bone mass, an earlier diagnosis can now be made before the fractures occur. Histomorphometry of bone biopsy specimens show a decrease in total bone volume and reduction in trabecular and to a lesser extent cortical bone due to a parallel loss of osteoid and mineral components. Thin trabeculae with normal osteoid and normal mineralization result.

Osteomalacia: Decreased mineralization of bone associated with an increased unmineralized osteoid.

Osteitis fibrosa: Increased parathyroid hormone-mediated osteoclastic bone resorption with replacement of normal bone by fibrous tissue.

Trabecular bone: Is the type of bone with the greatest surface area and metabolic activity, while cortical (or osteoidal) bone is much less active in remodeling.

There are multiple systemic and local factors that affect bone metabolism through either a negative or positive effect on bone resorption or formation. These have been summarized by Raisz.

(+ = increase, − = decrease, ( ) = indirect mechanism.)

	Resorption	*Formation*
1. Calcium regulating hormones		
PTH (parathyroid hormone)	+	+
1,25-dihydroxyvitamin D	+	−
calcitonin	−	no effect
2. Systemic hormones		
growth hormone	no effect	(+)
glucocorticoids	(+)	−
thyroid hormones	+	+
insulin	no effect	+
estrogens	(−)	(−)
3. Local factors		
prostaglandin E_2	+	+
interleukin-1	+	−,(+)
interferon-alpha	−	−
insulin-like growth factor	no effect	+
transforming growth factor-beta	−,(+)	+

The local and systemic milieu and other factors like degree of muscle activity, effect of gravity, exercise, etc. are also important. Abnormalities in the circulating (endogenous or exogenous) hormones or local concentration of any of these hormones and autacoids can result in decreased or unmineralized bone mass. Below is a brief review of some of these conditions, their diagnosis and therapy.

OSTEOPOROSIS

A decrease in total bone mass can occur as a primary or secondary disorder. Regardless of the etiology, the clinical risks are the same—frequent fractures with minimal or no trauma.

The proportion of cortical and trabecular bone varies between bones and between areas of bone. For example, vertebral bodies consist of approximately 70% trabecular and 30% cortical bone. The intertrochanteric area of the femur is composed of equal parts of trabecular and cortical bones. In general, the diaphysis of all bones is mostly (over 90%) cortical bone, while the metaphysis has more trabecular bone (about 25%). Because of their composition, the vertebrae, the distal radius, and the femoral neck are the most common sites of fracture in patients with osteoporosis, but the pelvis, the ribs, and the proximal humerus may also be involved.

Classification of osteoporosis

1. Primary
   a) Type I or post-menopausal
   b) Type II or senile
2. Secondary
   a) corticosteroid-induced
   b) in association with hypoestrogenic amenorrhea from any cause (e.g., hyperprolactinemia, excessive athletic activity, anorexia nervosa, etc.)
   c) prolonged bed rest
   d) thyroid hormone excess (usually iatrogenic) produces a hypercalciuric effect and increased bone resorption and formation
   e) multiple myeloma
   f) others

1. *Primary Osteoporosis (POP)*
   Type I or post-menopausal osteoporosis is due to the rapid decline in bone mass that occurs following loss of estrogenic hormones at menopause. It is more common in white and Asian women than in black women. The mechanism by which race imparts a protective effect to blacks compared to whites may be the ability of the black skeleton to achieve a higher peak bone mass as well as its much lower rate of bone turnover (about 35% of the rate in whites). Normal women lose bone at the rate of 0.3 to 1% a year after age 30-40. This increases to about 5% yearly during the first five years after menopause. Patients tend to develop spontaneous vertebral crush fractures and distal radial fractures from minimal trauma.

   Type II or senile osteoporosis occurs in both sexes, usually after age 70, but affects women worse because by this age, their total bone mass has already decreased substantially. Both groups are more susceptible to spontaneous vertebral wedge fractures and hip fractures from low impact falls. Over 90% of all hip fractures occur in the over 70 age group with reported mortalities of 30% and similar rates of nursing home placement.

Several epidemiologic factors appear to increase the risk for osteoporosis, including smoking, excessive alcohol intake, early age at menopause, immobilization (can cause 5% loss of bone calcium per month), little exposure to sunlight, diabetes, and positive family history. In contrast, increased body size is protective.

The role of specific calcium hormones, systemic hormones, and local factors in the pathogenesis of POP is not completely elucidated. While low levels of active vitamin D in this age group are well-documented, a well-designed double-blind prospective trial with calcitriol for two years did not show efficacy (in fact, although not statistically significant, the group on calcitriol had 25% new fractures compared to 16% in the placebo group). Likewise, although increased levels of parathyroid hormone have been found in patients with POP, patients in the 50-70 age group with primary hyperparathyroidism do not appear to be at increased risk of vertebral fractures, so the elevated PTH is unlikely to be a major culprit.

Diagnosis

Serum chemistries are normal in these patients, including serum calcium and phosphorus and alkaline phosphatase. If anemia, or an elevated sedimentation rate are present, multiple myeloma should be excluded by obtaining a serum protein electrophoresis, and Bence Jones protein in the urine. Patients on thyroid replacement should have their thyroxine and TSH levels checked and be kept on the lowest dose that maintains euthyroidism. The gold standard would be histomorphometric study of bone biopsy with double tetracycline labeling to be able to assess bone remodeling rate. However, a special bone lab is needed to process the specimen and interpret the findings, and obtaining an adequate specimen (from the iliac crest usually) is invasive and painful. Diagnosis in the preclinical or pre-osteopenic (by radiography) stage is limited by the sensitivity and specificity of the available methods. The preferred method is the single photon absorptiometry of the radius. It appears to correlate best with bone mineral content (BMC) overall. In addition, it works better for populations than for individual patients, and correlation with the sites of greatest interest (hip and vertebrae) is not as good as with overall BMC. Multiple other methods have been described, including dual photon absorptiometry and computed tomography.

An even more important question than which method to choose is how useful are these determinations in otherwise well patients (except as part of a study protocol). We agree with the 1987 American College of Physicians' position that the widespread application of these methods to screen for osteoporosis is premature.

Treatment

Multiple agents have been tried and variously reported to reduce bone loss, increase bone mass, or reduce fractures. Most are in agreement that prevention is more effective than treatment once fractures occur. All risk factors that can be modified should be, e.g., smoking, drinking, etc. In addition, achieving a high peak bone mass in the second and third decade is important. The current U.S. trend among young children and young adults to drink cola beverages rather than milk may lead to worsening risk of osteoporosis in the future. Cola beverages have a high phosphate content and replace one of the best traditional sources of dietary calcium. In the U.S., most women have an inadequate calcium intake. High intake of protein and phosphate both have a strong hypercalciuric effect. Calcium studies suggest an intake of 1000-1500 mg q.d. as necessary. Vitamin D from diet and sun exposure is usually sufficient. Encourage walking as a life-long habit. Restrict use of corticosteroids to conditions in which they clearly help and give for as short a period of time and as low a dose as will be effective; prevent or treat hypoestrogenic states.

1. *Estrogens* have been found to decrease the rate of bone loss of both trabecular and cortical bone following menopause. This effect occurs at very low doses (0.3 mg/day), although higher doses may produce an even better effect (0.625 to 1.25 mg conjugated estrogens per day). In addition, the risk of post-menopausal fractures of the vertebrae, hip and distal forearm is decreased by 50%. The effect is less marked but present at older ages.

   Although the effects of estrogen on bone were thought to be indirect, estrogen receptors in bone have now been found. Estrogens also have a protective effect against heart disease and have not been associated with a greater risk of thromboembolic complications or risk of breast cancer. Unopposed estrogen does increase the risk of endometrial hyperplasia and cancer to 750 per 100,000 with a 1% mortality. To decrease this risk, added progestins in a cyclical dose has been advocated. This produces return of the premenstrual syndrome (PMS) in susceptible individuals and withdrawal bleeding, which many patients do not tolerate. In addition, the long term cardiovascular risk of prolonged administration of progestins is unknown by may be significant. Daily continuous low dose progestin plus conjugated estrogens may successfully avoid menses and PMS. (Conjugated estrogen 0.625 mg q.d. plus medroxy-progesterone 2.5 mg q.d.)

WARNING: Estrogens are contra-indicated in any patient with a personal history of gynecologic or breast cancer. A family history of these cancers should be considered a relative contraindication.

2. *Calcium* supplementation by itself may have a minor effect in decreasing rate of loss from cortical (but not trabecular) bone. It does not have any proven preventive effect on fractures. Supplements are ususally given with estrogens. Any of the available calcium preparations are 30-40% absorbed if the patient has normal gastric acidity. If not, a soluble preparation may be preferred. An 8-ounce glass of milk contains approximately 200 mg of calcium.
3. *Fluoride* has been used but has a very high incidence of side effects (about 50%), mostly GI and rheumatic. The bone produced may be brittle if given without sufficient calcium. A slow release form with only a 16% incidence of side effects (25 mg b.i.d.) in combination (but not given simultaneously) with 1500 mg Ca q.d. and low dose vitamin D for three months every five months recently reported by Pak and colleagues appears efficacious. The findings await confirmation.
4. *Exercise* Low impact exercise (walking is ideal) for 30-40 minutes three to four times a week is useful in providing the stimulus for bone remodeling.
5. *Other agents* Calcitonin appears promising, especially in intranasal preparation of salmon calcitonin. Anabolic steroids (i.e., nandrolone decanoate) also appears useful, but more experience is needed.

   Finally, some non-steroidals (e.g., flurbiprofen) appear to have beneficial effects on the bone loss of periodontal disease and may prove beneficial to the whole skeleton, but this awaits further trials.

GLUCOCORTICOID-INDUCED OSTEOPOROSIS

Glucocorticoids interfere with intestinal calcium transport—possibly through the inhibition of synthesis of a carrier protein. Through a direct effect on bone, they inhibit bone matrix (collagen) and formation of osteoblast precursors. They also cause hypercalciuria.

Patients at risk for osteoporosis are usually those who have taken 10 mg of prednisone (or equivalent) for longer than three months, or total steroid dose greater than 30 gm of prednisone or its equivalent, age older than 50 years, and postmenopausal state. Irrespective of underlying disease, glucocorticoid treatment increases the risk of bone fractures, and alternate day therapy does not decrease the risk.

The currently recommended treatment includes supplemental calcium 500-1,000 mg/day, and vitamin D 50,000 IU one to two times per week. In women, estrogen (plus progestin) is also added. How effective this regimen is, is unclear (see above). However, close monitoring of serum and urine calcium (every 1-2 months and 4-6 months respectively) is needed to prevent potential complications.

OSTEOMALACIA

The hallmark of osteomalacia is abnormal or deficient mineralization of bone from primary or secondary vitamin D deficiency or from loss of calcium and phosphate. By bone biopsy, there is an increase in osteoid and a decrease in mineralization. These patients may complain for years of achiness and periarticular tenderness suggestive of fibromyalgia. By the time diagnostic serum chemistries are abnormal (low calcium, low phosphorus, and increased alkaline phosphatase) or radiographs reveal "looser zones" or "pseudofractures," the disease has been long-standing. In children, the equivalent syndrome is rickets.

An overview of the causes of osteomalacia are listed below.

1. Vitamin D deficiency
    a. Inadequate intake and reduced sunlight exposure
    b. Drug-induced catabolism of vitamin D (e.g., phenobarbital or phenytoin)
    c. Intestinal malabsorption

   d. Hepatic disease
   e. Renal disease with decreased 1,25 vitamin D production
2. Phosphate-wasting syndrome
   a. Acquired renal tubular defects with phosphate loss (so-called vitamin D-resistant rickets)
   b. Combined tubular defects (Fanconi's syndrome)
   c. Renal tubular acidosis
3. Mineralization defects

Treatment depends on adequate replacement of the vitamin or correction of the abnormal state.

OSTEITIS FIBROSA

This is a histologic diagnosis based on increased bone resorption and fibrous tissue replacement of the resorbed bone. It is due to excess parathyroid hormone (PTH), which induces an increase in mineral and matrix resorption. The serum calcium may be high and the serum phosphorus low. Serum PTH is elevated. The causes of osteitis fibrosa are listed below.

1. Primary hyperparathyroidism
2. Secondary hyperparathyroidism
   a. Vitamin D deficiency states
   b. "Primary" decrease in intestinal calcium absorption (e.g., with age)
   c. Reduced renal mass, such as in chronic renal failure

Treatment may require parathyroidectomy.

PAGET'S DISEASE OF BONE

This is a disease of unknown etiology (possibly viral) that produces striking radiographic changes of sclerosis, lytic activity, or both, usually associated with elevated serum alkaline phosphatase. Most patients are asymptomatic, but the lesions can resemble metastatic disease. Multicentric osteogenic sarcoma may occur in less than 1% of patients. Treatment with a NSAID is usually sufficient, but if it is not, biphosphonates or calcitonin can provide marked improvement.

SUGGESTED READINGS

1. Ott SM, Chestnut CH III. Calcitriol treatment is not effective in postmenopausal osteoporosis. Ann Intern Med. 1989; 110:267-74.

2. Raisz LG. Local and systemic factors in the pathogenesis of osteoporosis. N Engl J Med. 1988; 318:818-28.

3. Sewell KL. Modern therapeutic approaches to osteoporosis. Rheum Clin Dis North Am. 1989; 15:583-614.

Chapter 39

Vasculitis

The non-infectious vasculitides are a group of diseases whose pathology is characterized by inflammation and often necrosis of blood vessels. The ultimate result of the inflammatory process can be ischemia of the organs supplied by the involved vessels. These diseases are classified in several ways: (1) Clinically by organ systems involved and prognosis; (2) pathologically, by size of vessel involved by vasculitis and by the presence or absence of granulomas; (3) by differing immunologic mechanism; (4) by therapeutic approach. Vasculitis may be the only manifestation of an illness or it may be part of another primary illness such as systemic lupus erythematosus or a malignancy. Whatever the cause, the severity of the vasculitis depends to a large extent upon whether critical organ systems are involved and upon the responsiveness of the vascular inflammation to therapy.

CLASSIFICATION OF VASCULITIS ACCORDING TO VESSEL SIZE

1. Small Vessel Vasculitis:

   Hypersensitivity vasculitis
   Henoch-Schönlein purpura
   Vasculitis associated with connective tissue diseases:
      Rheumatoid vasculitis
      Lupus vasculitis
      Essential mixed cryoglobulinemia with vasculitis
      Sjögren's syndrome
      Serum sickness and serum sickness-like reactions
   Vasculitis associated with malignancies

2. Medium Vessel Necrotizing Vasculitis:

   Classical polyarteritis nodosa
   Wegener's granulomatosis
   Churg-Strauss allergic granulomatosis
   Systemic necrotizing vasculitis

3. Large Vessel Vasculitis

   Giant cell (temporal) arteritis
   Takayasu's arteritis

ETIOLOGY

The etiology of vasculitis is known in only a small percentage of patients. In general, it is felt that there may be many inciting agents capable of causing the same clinical symptoms in a susceptible host. One mechanism of inducing vasculitis is via immune complexes. A foreign antigen enters the circulation and stimulates antibody production, which in certain cases can lead to the establishment of circulating immune complexes. These complexes injure vessels by activating complement components and by stimulating other inflammatory mediators and chemotactic factors which attract polymorphonuclear cells. These cells release lysosomal enzymes which then damage the vessel wall.

The granulomatous vasculitides, on the other hand, are thought to be incited by antigenic stimulation of sensitized lymphocytes which then activate macrophages. These macrophages ultimately transform into epithelioid cells and later form granulomas. Vessel wall damage again occurs with release of lysosomal enzymes. In polyarteritis nodosa (PAN), a small to medium size vessel vasculitis, hepatitis B has been found to play an etiologic role, presumably secondary to circulating immune complexes of hepatitis B antigens and antibodies. HbsAg has been demonstrated in 10-54% of patients with PAN. Other factors, such as intravenous drug abuse (especially methamphetamine), acute viral illnesses causing acute serous otitis media, and, perhaps, chronic antigenic stimulation via desensitization for allergies have been implicated in the etiology of vasculitis.

In the hypersensitivity group of vasculitides, antibiotic drugs, such as penicillin and sulfa, and bacterial infections, such as beta-hemolytic streptococcus, are thought to induce immune complex formation and thereby elicit vasculitis. Endogenous sources such as tumors are felt to mediate the disease in a similar fashion. Each individual's unique immune response to an antigenic stimulus determines the type and severity of the vasculitis.

MAKING THE DIAGNOSIS

1. Vasculitis should be suspected in patients who have the clinical presentation of multiple organ system disease, such as rash, arthritis, pulmonary infiltrates, peripheral neuropathy, central nervous system symptoms, renal disease, or other organ involvement. The differential diagnosis of vasculitis and multi-organ involvement include diseases such as bacterial endocarditis, atrial myxomas, and cholesterol emboli in patients who have recently undergone a catheterization procedure, so these conditions must be excluded.
2. The diagnosis is confirmed pathologically by biopsy of the involved organ and finding the presence of inflammation within blood vessel walls. The most commonly biopsied tissues are skin, nerve, lung, kidney, and muscle. If the involved organ systems are not amenable to biopsy, the diagnosis may sometimes be confirmed by finding evidence suggestive of inflammation in the blood vessels on angiogram. For hypersensitivity vasculitis, the finding of leukocytoclastic changes (debris from nuclei of polymorphonuclear leukocytes) on skin biopsy is sufficient to make the diagnosis. To diagnose medium vessel vasculitis, it is helpful to biopsy tissue other than skin (nerve, muscle, or lung) to get larger vessels on the tissue. In polyarteritis nodosa, multiple microaneurysms at bifurcations of the hepatic, splenic, or renal arteries can be demonstrated by arteriography.

   The presence of certain autoantibodies (anti-neutrophil cytoplasmic antibody and lymphocytotoxins) as a way to diagnose Wegener's and related vasculitides appears very promising and is available in some commercial laboratories.
3. To diagnose a specific type of vasculitis, one must recognize certain clinical patterns of organ involvement and correlate them with the patient in question. *Wegener's granulomatosis* classically involves the upper and lower respiratory tract, kidneys, and nerves. *Polyarteritis*, in contrast, rarely involves the lungs but commonly affects skin,

nerves, kidneys and gastrointestinal tract. *Churg-Strauss allergic granulomatosis* most often occurs in patients with a prior history of atopy and severe asthma, and presents with eosinophilia, pulmonary and renal insufficiency, severe hypertension, gastrointestinal bleeding, and even death, if not diagnosed and treated early and aggressively.

Hypersensitivity vasculitis is a disease primarily of small vessels (post capillary venules) whose major manifestation is cutaneous involvement characterized as palpable purpura. Although other organ systems can be involved, it is usually mild and rarely causes severe organ dysfunction.

Large vessel vasculitis is seen in two diseases involving quite different patient populations, *temporal (giant cell) arteritis* and *Takayasu's arteritis*. Temporal arteritis classically affects patients over the age of 50. Local symptoms are temporal headaches, visual changes progressing to total blindness, and jaw claudication. Patients can be quite ill with fever, weight loss, malaise, and proximal myalgias. The arteries affected are usually branches of the external carotid artery although occasionally intracranial arteries can be involved. This type of vasculitis, of which blindness is its most feared complication, responds well to steroids (see Chapter 40).

Takayasu's arteritis, also known as pulseless disease, affects young women of Japanese ancestry. The vessels primarily affected include the aorta and its branches (carotid and subclavian arteries). Ultimately, inflammation occludes the lumens of these arteries, thereby compromising blood flow to the head and extremities. The course of Takayasu's arteritis is variable, making assessment of therapy difficult. However, it is generally recognized that the response to steroids in this disease is not as good as in temporal arteritis.

COMPLICATIONS OF VASCULITIS

Serious complications of vasculitis include pulmonary and renal insufficiency, hypertension and its sequelae, and permanent neurological deficits.

Renal involvement is common in both polyarteritis nodosa and Wegener's granulomatosis and can be a cause of death in both diseases. *Hypertension,* developing as a complication of vasculitis, may further contribute to progressive renal functional loss.

Peripheral neuropathy is seen in 60-70% of patients with PAN, and *cerebral* manifestations are almost equally as common. Unfortunately, in patients with *mononeuritis multiplex*, there is often incomplete recovery from ischemic lesions of the vasa nervorum. Some residual permanent weakness and numbness may remain, usually affecting nerves originating from the sacral plexus. Acutely, food drop may result in deep venous thromboses because of inability to move the food and ankle adequately. Although Wegener's granulomatosis also has peripheral nerve involvement, optic and other *cranial nerve* involvement is more commonly seen due to direct nerve injury from contiguous granulomatous disease. Remissions of neurological involvement in Wegener's granulomatosis occur often as the disease is treated.

Acute abdominal complications secondary to intra-abdominal arteritis have been reported in PAN and SLE. Neurological involvement and thrombocytopenia are common accompaniments in patients with PAN who have abdominal involvement. Clinical problems resulting from necrotizing arteritis in the abdomen are bowel necrosis, perforation with resultant peritonitis, and ruptured intrahepatic and intra-renal aneurysms. Bowel infarction presents insidiously with few findings except occult or frank blood in the stool. The patient has often been on steroids before, and the abdominal findings may be quite masked. A high index or suspicion is required to make the diagnosis before a catastrophic peritonitis ensues.

TREATMENT AND PROGNOSIS

Treatment is dependent upon the type of vasculitis identified. The first, most obvious treatment is to treat or remove any known inciting agent. For the less severe, small vessel hypersensitivity vasculitides restricted to only a few organ systems, e.g., skin, joints, and gastrointestinal tract, no other treatment may be necessary. On the other hand, untreated Wegener's granulomatosis has a mortality of 95% at five years, and most untreated polyarteritis nodosa patients are dead within one year. Fortunately, therapy with cytotoxic agents, particularly cyclophosphamide, has greatly improved survival in these diseases. The reports that some cases of Wegener's granulomatosis may respond to trimethoprim-sulfamethoxazole is an exciting development that awaits further confirmation.

In addition to medium vessel vasculitides, small vessel vasculitis, such as that seen in rheumatoid arthritis and systemic lupus, can be fatal if not treated with steroids and/or cyclophosphamide. The recommended dose of cyclophosphamide is 1-2 mg/kg of body weight per day. Attempts should be made to keep the neutrophil count between 1000 to 1500/mm^3. If there is no favorable therapeutic response within two weeks, the daily dose can be slowly increased (by 25-mg increments every 2-3 weeks) until a response is obtained or toxicity (leukopenia or hematuria) occurs. For patients with acute fulminant disease, steroids should be added at 1-2 mg/kg/day, in divided doses for their immediate anti-inflammatory effect.

COMPLICATIONS OF TREATMENT

The most frequent complications of treatment of these diseases with steroids and cyclophosphamide are *infection* and *malignancy*. The risk of infection, especially from opportunistic organisms such as *Pneumocystis carinii* or cytomegalovirus, is high and requires close surveillance for presence of recurrent fever or depressed white blood cell counts. Although cyclophosphamide can cause fibrosis or even cancer of the bladder, this side effect can be minimized by generous fluid intake during the day to dilute the toxic metabolites of the drug or by giving monthly "pulse" treatments rather than daily doses. Lymphoproliferative malignancies are another long-term risk of cyclophosphamide and other cytotoxic agents (see Chapter 45). Almost certain death from life-threatening vasculitis makes the risk of drug toxicity acceptable.

SUGGESTED READINGS

1. Duffy J, Lidsky, MD, Sharp JT, et al. Polyarthritis, polyarteritis, and hepatitis B. Medicine. 1987; 55:19-37.

2. Fan PT, Davis JA, Somer R, Kaplan K, Bluestone R. A clinical approach to systemic vasculitis. Sem Arthritis Rheum. 1980; 9:249-304.

3. Fauci AS, Haynes BF, Katz P, Wolff SM. Wegener's granulomatosis: Prospective clinical and therapeutic experience with 85 patients for 21 years. Ann Intern Med. 1983; 98:76-85.

4. Scott DGI, Bacon PA. Intravenous cyclophosphamide plus methylprednisolone in treatment of systemic rheumatoid vasculitis. Am J Med. 1984; 76:377-384.

5. Wolf SM, Fauci AS, Katz P, Haynes BF. Cyclophosphamide therapy of severe necrotizing vasculitis. N Eng J Med. 1979; 31:235-238.

6. Lie JT. Classification and immunodiagnosis of vasculitis: A new solution or promises unfulfilled? J Rheumatol. 1988; 15:728-32.

Chapter 40

Polymyalgia Rheumatica and Giant Cell (Temporal) Arteritis

The relationship between polymyalgia rheumatica (PMR) and temporal arteritis (TA) is well established. Epidemiologic studies in this country report:

—50% of patients with TA have PMR
—10 to 20% of patients with PMR have symptomatic TA
—the range of patients with PMR reported to have occult ("silent") TA is 5-50%.

The basis for the relationship between these two clinical syndromes remains controversial. Although PMR and TA affect similar populations (over age 55, with a female to male ratio of 2:1), their coexpression is more frequent than expected from chance alone. Most investigators believe PMR and TA represent a spectrum of disease with a common underlying immune mechanism.

POLYMYALGIA RHEUMATICA (PMR)

PMR is a vague constellation of systemic and musculoskeletal symptoms that may occur (1) as an isolated clinical syndrome, (2) associated with occult or symptomatic temporal arteritis, or (3) as a manifestation of occult infection, neoplasm, or other connective tissue disease.

A. CLINICAL FINDINGS
   1. PMR is rarely seen in patients under the age of 50, and most are older than 65.

2. Pain and stiffness of proximal muscle groups is characteristic. Weakness, if present, is only a minor component and helps distinguish PMR from polymyositis.
3. Onset of symptoms is usually insidious (over weeks) with shoulder girdle muscles involved more frequently than pelvic girdle muscles. A subgroup of patients may present with very abrupt onset of symptoms.
4. Morning stiffness and "gelling" phenomenon are common (similar or rheumatoid arthritis). In fact, differentiating RA from PMR of acute onset in some patients may be quite difficult.
5. Systemic symptoms are common and occur early, including fever and sweats, fatigue and malaise, anorexia and weight loss. In these patients, occult TA is more likely to be present.
6. Spontaneous remission may occur in three months to three years, but in some patients, symptoms persist longer.

B. LABORATORY FINDINGS
1. Erythrocyte sedimentation rate (ESR) is almost always elevated (and frequently markedly elevated) in both PMR and TA. Other non-specific abnormalities in both PMR and TA are anemia and elevated alkaline phosphatase.
2. Muscle enzymes, EMGs and muscle biopsies are usually normal or have non-specific changes.

C. TREATMENT
1. PMR, when not complicated by TA, will respond rapidly to either NSAIDs or *low dose* (10-15 mg per day) prednisone.
2. If symptoms persist and the ESR had not decreased on this therapy after three or four weeks, you should
   a. look for an "occult" temporal arteritis with temporal artery biopsies,
   b. consider other potential diagnoses like rheumatoid arthritis, infection, or paraneoplastic syndrome.
3. Remember that PMR is a self-remitting condition and therapy should be continued only as long as necessary to treat the symptoms.

TEMPORAL ARTERITIS

A. CLINICAL FINDINGS

Temporal arteritis, also known as cranial arteritis, is a form of giant cell-arteritis (GCA) that occurs primarily in the elderly. If untreated,

10-50% of patients with TA will develop permanent, partial, or complete blindness. Like PMR, TA is a self-remitting disease. If appropriately treated (see below), recurrences of TA are unusual after the first six months; however, in some patients, the disease remains active or recurs over longer periods.

Clinical Manifestations	*Frequency (%)*
—Headache (new onset or change in pattern or intensity, often in the temporal or occipital area)	60
—Tender, swollen, nodular temporal artery	55
—Pulseless temporal artery	50
—Constitutional symptoms presenting as a fever of unknown etiology (fever, malaise, weight loss)	50
—Visual symptoms (blurring, diplopia, amaurosis fugax, and partial or complete blindness)	40
—Jaw claudication	35
—Facial pain (including tongue)	20
—Depression	20

Although known as temporal or cranial arteritis, the vascular inflammation may involve other large arteries. Fatal acute aortic dissection secondary to TA has been described.

B. LABORATORY FINDINGS

1. The non-specific findings of anemia, markedly elevated ESR and increased alkaline phosphatase are common to both PMR and TA
2. The diagnosis of TA should *always* be confirmed by a temporal artery biopsy. This is because other conditions can mimic TA (e.g., atherosclerosis, polyarteritis, or tumor). The classic pathologic changes on biopsy are those of *granulomatous arteritis* with prominent Langhans' giant cells in areas of disruption of the internal elastic lamina of the arterial wall. Biopsies obtained within 3-5 days of starting steroids should still show typical changes. Beyond this time, changes may be less specific.
3. The lesions of TA may occur in a "skip" pattern, so that multiple sections of the biopsied artery should be examined. The biopsy should be made of the tender or nodular area of the ar-

tery. If the artery is not clinically abnormal, the biopsy should be generous (5-6 cm) and examined in its entirety to improve chances of detecting the arteritis.

4. If the biopsy of one temporal artery is normal but the suspicion of TA remains high, the contralateral temporal artery should also be biopsied. If both temporal artery biopsies are adequately examined and found to be normal, other diagnostic considerations should be re-examined.

C. TREATMENT

Due to the significant risk of blindness from TA, corticosteroids (prednisone 60-80 mg per day) should be initiated as soon as a presumptive diagnosis of TA is made. The temporal artery biopsy should be performed immediately or within 24-48 hours of beginning steroids (pathology may become "nondiagnostic" after short periods of steroid therapy). A typical course of prednisone for uncomplicated TA would progress as follows:

Weeks	*Daily Prednisone Dose (mg)*
1 through 4	60 (may initially be given in divided doses for greater anti-inflammatory effect, then consolidated to an early AM dose)
4-6	50
6-8	40
8-16	decrease by 5 mg every two weeks
16-24	decrease by 2.5 mg every two weeks
24-52	maintain steroid dose between 10 and 25 mg

An alternative would be to add a NSAID after the first six months of prednisone therapy and taper the patient off the prednisone more rapidly. This is particularly appropriate for patients at greater risk of steroid toxicity (e.g., those with hypertension, diabetes, cataracts, severe osteoporosis or atherosclerosis). In patients with severe side effects from steroids, azathioprine in doses of 1.5-2.5 mg/kg per day has provided anti-inflammatory control and steroid sparing.

Close monitoring of therapy is required due to the dire consequences of TA, the elderly population being treated, and the potential toxicity of corticosteroids. Monthly evaluations for the first half year of therapy should include review of symptoms of PMR and TA, physical examination, and ESR.

The decision to increase the corticosteroid dose during the tapering course should be based on the recurrence of TA symptoms (important to distinguish these from PMR symptoms!) rather than changes in ESR levels. However, rising ESR levels should increase vigilance for possible relapse. Alternate day steroids are usually insufficient to treat temporal arteritis in the early stages, but may be tried after the first 4-6 months for more rapid taper.

SUGGESTED READINGS

1. Huston KA, Hunder GG, Lie JT, et al. Temporal arteritis: A 25-year epidemiologic, clinical and pathologic study. Ann Intern Med. 1978; 88:162.

2. Hunder GG, Sheps SG, Allen GL, Joyce JW. Daily and alternate-day corticosteroid regimens in treatment of giant cell arteritis. Ann Intern Med. 1975; 82:613-18.

3. Hunder GG, Michet CJ. Giant cell arteritis and polymyalgia rheumatica. Clin Rheum Dis. 1985; 11:471-83.

Chapter 41

Rheumatic Diseases and the Skin

The skin is often a target organ in the connective tissue diseases. This chapter is an overview of skin lesions often associated with rheumatic disease.

URTICARIA AND RELATED LESIONS

True urticaria and urticarial-like lesions may occur in patients with connective tissue diseases. The differential of urticaria and urticarial-like lesions includes:

1. *Chronic idiopathic* urticaria, which can be quite difficult to treat. As the name implies, its etiology is often unknown.
2. *Hypocomplementemic vasculitis* has been reported in middle-aged women with recurrent urticaria, arthralgias and arthritis, abdominal pain, mild renal disease, and a low frequency of ANA positivity. Serologically, the illness is characterized by depressed levels of total complement and elevated levels of circulating immune complexes.

   Histologically it is characterized as a leucocytoclastic vasculitis, except for 10 to 15% who have mild mononuclear infiltrates rather than polymorphonuclear infiltration and lysis. There may be positive staining for immunoglobulins and complement at the dermal epidermal junction and within the blood vessels. It has been reported that these patients may develop a late-stage, life-threatening, obstructive lung disease although it is not clear what contribution long-term cigarette smoking has in these patients.
3. *Urticaria associated with connective tissue diseases* occurs primarily in Sjögren's syndrome and systemic lupus erythematosus. One study

reported 40% of patients with primary Sjögren's syndrome had urticaria, and in these patients hypocomplementemic vasculitis and antibodies to SS-A/Ro were frequently seen. In systemic lupus erythematosus, 5 to 15% will have urticaria. The urticaria has a predilection for the trunk, arms, palms, and soles of the feet, persists for over 24 hours, and frequently heals with residual hyperpigmentation. It is usually seen in the setting of SLE patients who have active systemic disease and low serum complement values. Histologically, leucocytoclastic vasculitis is seen in 70 to 80% and mononuclear infiltrates in 12 to 20%.

4. *Urticaria* can also be seen *in association with infection*, e.g., hepatitis B infection, occurring in 10 to 20% of prodomal cases. It may precede clinical jaundice by 2 to 30 days, is often associated with cryoglobulinemia, and is characterized by deposits of fibrin, C3, IgM, and hepatitis B surface antigen in the skin. Urticaria may also present in association with infectious mononucleosis and serum sickness.

SWEET'S SYNDROME (ACUTE FEBRILE NEUTROPHILIC DERMATOSIS)

Sweet's syndrome is characterized by the abrupt onset of very painful red plaques on the arms, face, and neck. Histologically it is characterized by dense dermal infiltration by mature polymorphonuclear leukocytes. Clinically, there is fever and neutrophilia, arthralgias, and arthritis. A good response is often seen with corticosteroids, and the lesions are usually non-scarring. Sweet's syndrome recurs in 30% of patients, is usually idiopathic, but may occur in association with an underlying myeloproliferative disorder, which should be looked for in patients with this condition.

EOSINOPHILIC FASCIITIS

Eosinophilic fasciitis is characterized by the skin of the extremities becoming taut, indurated, and often, painful. There is a history of increased physical exertion of the affected area in around 50% of cases. Although it is often said to be a scleroderma variant, there is no associated Raynaud's phenomenon or visceral involvement and no distal involvement of the digits. Peripheral eosinophilia is seen in 30 to 40% in association with hypergammaglobulinemia and an elevated sedimentation rate. Approximately 10% of patients with eosinophilic fasciitis will have a hematologic abnormality such as aplastic anemia. Isolated thrombocytopenia and leukemia have also been reported. In order to make the diagnosis, a deep biopsy of skin and subcutaneous tissue to the fascial level needs to be performed. On deep biopsy, there is a diffuse infiltrate of lymphocytes, plasma cells, and eosinophils in the subcutaneous tissue near the thickened fibrotic fascia. The natural history of this condition is unknown but is thought to be responsive to corticosteroids in most instances.

ERYTHEMA NODOSUM

Erythema nodosum is characterized by the sudden appearance of crops of tender, painful erythematous and slightly raised nodules, usually occurring on the leg, below the knee, around the ankles and dorsum of the foot, but not on the soles of the feet. Erythema nodosum may also occur on the extensor surfaces of the lower arm. These lesions reach their maximum size of 0.5 to 2 cm in diameter in a day and they last usually one to three weeks, in which time the lesions pass through color changes including yellow, green, and blue and resemble bruises. When they resolve, they leave no permanent pigmentary changes and are non-scarring. Pathologically, erythema nodosum appears to be a septal panniculitis. In contrast, Weber-Christian is associated with a lobular panniculitis.

Erythema nodosum (EN) is often idiopathic but may also be associated with a number of conditions, including tuberculosis, sarcoidosis, streptococcal infections, inflammatory bowel disease, fungal infections, drugs, and leprosy. EN due to tuberculosis usually occurs within three to eight weeks after the primary infection. The association of EN with bilateral hilar adenopathy and arthritis from sarcoidosis is known as Lofgren's syndrome. Erythema nodosum may occur with rheumatic fever and acute glomerulonephritis with usually only two or three lesions present at one time. In inflammatory bowel disease, EN may occur in association with flares of bowel disease and is usually improved with control of the bowel inflammation. Skin complications occur in approximately 10% of cases of ulcerative colitis, 25% of those with peripheral joint involvement, and 5% of those with spondylitis.

EN is primarily seen in association with coccidiomycosis and histoplasmosis, and is rare in North American blastomycosis. It has also been associated with sulfa medications, penicillin, and oral contraceptives. In the erythema nodosum associated with leprosy, the skin lesions are usually associated with fever, orchitis, arthritis, lymphadenopathy, and polyneuritis.

Various forms of treatment have been tried for erythema nodosum, including salicylates, colchicine, and a number of the non-steroidals with variable benefits.

NODULES

Rheumatoid nodules occur in about 20% of patients with rheumatoid arthritis. They are usually on the extensor surfaces and pressure points and only rarely ulcerate. Surgical removal is not recommended as there is a marked tendency to recur.

Tophi also commonly develop over the extensor surfaces and can mimic rheumatoid nodules but usually have a more chalky appearance to them. If there is any question, a suspected tophus can be aspirated to determine whether urate crystals are present.

Nodules along tendons may also be seen in the hyperlipoproteinemias, particularly types II and IV which can also be associated with a pauci- or polyarthritis. The nodule responds to therapy for the hyperlipidemia. Skin papules and nodules may also be seen in chronic sarcoidosis and in Wegener's granulomatosis. Osler's nodes are characteristic of subacute bacterial endocarditis and are seen on the palms and the soles of the feet, but are increasingly uncommon in the antibiotic era.

RHEUMATIC ULCERS

Digital ulcers are frequently seen in severe Raynaud's phenomenon, particularly in association with connective tissue disease, most commonly scleroderma. Ulcerative lesions in the buttock area should raise the possibility of associated vasculitis. Ulcers in the lower extremities are often seen in rheumatoid arthritis, usually with associated vasculitis, in scleroderma, and in Sjögren's syndrome associated with an underlying vasculitis with or without cryoglobulinemia.

PYODERMA GANGRENOSUM

Pyoderma grangrenosum (PG) is an uncommon skin disorder first described in 1930 that first presents as a pustule that rapidly ulcerates and produces a characteristic burrowing ulcer with heaped-up purple borders. When these lesions heal, they form a cribriform scar. It is not considered a vasculitis although vascular damage has been reported in the erythematous border of the surrounding uninvolved skin. The etiology is unknown. As soon as the ulcer develops, secondary bacterial colonization of the necrotic area occurs, but the original lesion is always sterile.

Between 30-50% of the patients reported in the literature have no other associated conditions. In other patients, inflammatory bowel disease (especially ulcerative colitis) and polyarthritis (both classical seropositive RA and a seronegative erosive polyarthritis) are the most common. Recently, four patients with PG and polyarthritis were reported who had an intra-abdominal abscess secondary to a perforated diverticulum. Removal of the inflammatory segment of bowel resulted in complete resolution of the previously refractory PG lesions.

Another reported associated finding is an IgA paraproteinemia and/or myeloma. Effective treatment of the associated disease has been variously described as producing (or not) remission of PG. Steroids in high daily doses of 1-2 mg/kg prednisone are usually effective, but relapses are frequent during dose tapering. In some patients, the lesions are self-limited, while in others, additional agents may be tried with variable success, including colchicine 0.6 mg b.i.d. (if patient has normal renal function) or cytotoxic drugs. Although most lesions occur in the lower extremities, the trunk and upper extremities may also be involved. In some patients, onset of PG develops after surgery or trauma in the area involved. Antibiotics are only useful in the management of secondary infections. Skin grafts often fail and, in fact, may exacerbate the condition.

SUGGESTED READINGS

1. Schorr-Lesnick AB, Brandt LJ. Selected rheumatologic and dermatologic manifestations of inflammatory bowel disease. Am J Gastroenterol. 1988; 83:216-23.

2. Klein S, Mayer L, Present DH, et al. Extraintestinal manifestations in patients with diverticulitis. Ann Intern Med. 1988; 108:700-702.

Chapter 42

Rheumatic Diseases and the Eye

Connective tissue diseases, and sometimes the drugs used in their treatment, may affect any of the elements of the eye—from the cornea anteriorly to the retina and optic nerve posteriorly. Some rheumatic diseases affect certain portions of the eye with so much regularity that an overview of these conditions merits inclusion in a manual like this.

COMPONENTS OF THE EYE INVOLVED BY RHEUMATIC DISEASE

1. *Lacrimal glands.* Deficiency of aqueous layer is the cause for dry eyes in Sjögren's syndrome. However, other conditions associated with musculoskeletal symptoms like sarcoidosis may present with lacrimal gland enlargement. A differential diagnosis of lacrimal glands swelling and/or malfunction was discussed earlier (see Chapter 31).
2. *Ocular musculature.* An uncommon form of myasthenia gravis limited to the ocular muscles has been described secondary to D-penicillamine. The patient develops double vision a few months after beginning treatment at which time this complication should be suspected. Diagnosis is established by the classic response to Tensilon. Treatment with anticholinesterases and discontinuation of the second line agent are associated with improvement. Complete resolution may take several months to years.
3. *Ocular hypertension* (glaucoma) may develop secondary to chronic uveitis. The patient may see halos around lights.
4. *Refractive errors* have been reported with many of the non-steroidal anti-inflammatory drugs, but not every patient appears to be susceptible.

5. *Lens abnormalities*. Dislocation is seen in patients with Marfan's syndrome and other related conditions. Opacification of the lens—cataracts—are a well known complication of prolonged steroid treatment but may also develop and association with chronic or recurrent uveitis.
6. *Conjunctival inflammation*. When the conjunctiva alone is inflamed, the eye may hurt, but photophobia is not present (as opposed to uveitis, where contraction of the iris and ciliary body are associated with pain). Band keratopathy due to deposition of calcium on the cornea may also be associated with deposits in the conjunctiva and produce reddened conjunctivae and calcification and sensation of grittiness and pain in the eye. It is best diagnosed by slit-lamp examination and is associated with hypercalcemia (e.g., renal failure, sarcoidosis, hyperparathyroidism—all of which have rheumatic manifestations). Band keratopathy may also be seen in patients with JRA (juvenile RA) associated with chronic uveitis.
7. *Scleritis*, inflammation of the sclera, is common in RA and may also be involved in Wegener's granulomatosis and relapsing polychondritis. Thinning of the sclera leads to a bluish tinge of the eye associated with RA. Eventual necrosis and globe preformation may occur (scleromalacia perforans).
8. *Keratitis* (corneal inflammation). The characteristic punctate keratitis associated with Sjögren's syndrome (primary or secondary) is by far the most commonly seen corneal involvement.
9. *Uveitis*. The uveal tract consists of the iris, ciliary bodies, and choroid. Inflammation of the uveal tract can be divided into anterior and posterior uveitis. Anterior uveitis includes both iritis and iridocyclitis, that is, inflammation of the iris with or without associated involvement of the ciliary body. Posterior uveitis consists of choroiditis. Approximately 33% of patients presenting to an ophthalmology clinic with uveitis will have a rheumatic disease.

   Juvenile rheumatoid arthritis, the spondyloarthropathies (ankylosing spondylitis, psoriatic spondylitis, Reiter's syndrome, and gut-associated spondylitis), and sarcoidosis are all well-known causes (or associations) of uveitis. Relapsing polychondritis is a much less common cause.
10. *Retinal abnormalities* are most commonly seen in association with vasculitis. Blindness secondary to giant cell arteritis involvement of either the central retinal artery or, more commonly, branches

of the ophthalmic artery producing ischemia of the optic nerve is the most dreaded complication of this disease. Retinal vasculitis leading to more focal or patchy ischemia is characteristic of systemic lupus leading to the development of "cotton wool" spots. Antimalarials used to treat SLE or RA may also produce a retinopathy with a characteristic "bull's eye." It can be identified early by demonstrating red color blindness.

SPECIFIC EYE INVOLVEMENT IN RHEUMATIC DISEASES

Juvenile Rheumatoid Arthritis

Eye involvement occurs in 17 percent of JRA patients. The typical profile of a JRA patient with chronic iridocyclitis consists of: (1) a young girl (female-to-male ratio of 4:1); (2) early onset of disease, usually before the age of four; (3) mono- or pauciarticular involvement in 90 percent; (4) the onset of arthritis antedating eye involvement by 3 1/2 years; and (5) ANA positivity in 70-80 percent. Bilateral eye involvement occurs in 66 percent. There is no correlation between the activity of the joints and eyes. Often eye involvement persists while the arthritis is in remission. One of the most striking features of chronic iridocyclitis is the absence of symptoms or obvious signs of ocular inflammation Slit lamp examination is needed to search for eye involvement in JRA. Early treatment appears to decrease the frequency of JRA ocular complications such as cataracts (22-50%), band keratopathy (13-41%), and glaucoma. First line treatment consists of topical corticosteroids and mydriatics. Systemic corticosteroids may be required in resistant cases.

Regular ophthalmologic examinations are imperative in children with JRA, particularly those with pauciarticular involvement. Remember, the less the joints are involved, the more the eyes are involved. These patients should have an eye examination, including slit-lamp, every three months for five years, then every six months for seven years or to age 15. In patients with pauciarticular involvement, some would continue to monitor frequently through early adulthood. Patients with systemic or polyarticular involvement should be examined every six months for at least five years. Remember, it is better to examine too often than to miss asymptomatic iridocyclitis, especially since surgery for the ocular complications of iridocyclitis is not usually successful in preventing blindness.

Rheumatoid Arthritis (see also Chapter 26)

Unlike JRA, adult RA is not usually associated with iridocyclitis. The most common eye involvement is keratoconjunctivitis sicca, part of the sicca complex of Sjögren's syndrome. Other involvement is well described, including episcleritis, scleritis, scleromalacia perforans, and corneal melting.

Episcleritis is inflammation of the loose connective tissue between the conjunctiva and the sclera. It occurs in 0.17% of RA patients. It is mild, does not progress to scleritis, and usually does not need treatment. In only 5% of patients presenting to an eye clinic with episcleritis is there an associated connective tissue disease.

Scleritis occurs in 0.67% of RA patients and may either be focal, diffuse, or nodular. An associated uveitis may be present. Patients complain of a deep aching, and slit lamp examination is required for confirmation of scleritis. Scleral thinning may occur. Perforation may also occur, espcially if the scleritis is necrotizing. Aggressive treatment is usually necessary (topical corticosteroids are usually insufficient). Oral prostaglandin inhibitors, such as indomethacin, prednisone, and, occasionally, cyclophosphamide may be required.

Systemic Lupus Erythematosus

Retinal hemorrhage occurs in 5-28% and cotton wool spots in 6-28% of SLE patients. Cotton wool spots are small, fluffy, white exudates usually adjacent to arterioles and represent microinfarcts of the nerve fiber layer. The term cytoid body, often used interchangeably with cotton wool spot, is actually a histologic feature of the cotton wool spot and represents swelling of degenerating axial nerve fibers.

Ankylosing Spondylitis

Approximately 20-30% of patients with ankylosing spondylitis develop an acute nongranulomatous uveitis, usually an iritis. The back involvement usually starts first and there is no correction between the severity of the spondylitis and the eye disease. The iritis is usually unilateral, but moves from side to side. The eye is red and painful and patients complain of photophobia. The iritis usually is very responsive to topical steroids and mydriatics but has a tendency to recur. Approximately

50% of iritis patients are HLA-B27 positive and may represent a "forme fruste" of ankylosing spondylitis since many lack clinical or radiographic features of spondylitis.

Reiter's Syndrome

Eye involvement is usually a conjunctivitis and less commonly an iritis. It is difficult to obtain an accurate frequency of conjunctivitis in Reiter's because it is usually so mild that it escapes detection. Chronic iridocyclitis and optic neuritis have also been reported, but are rare.

Inflammatory Bowel Diseases

Acute iritis occurs in 11% of patients with ulcerative colitis, especially in association with spondylitis, and 2.4-5% of patients with Crohn's disease.

Psoriatic Arthritis

In one reported study, conjunctivitis occurred in 20%, uveitis in 10%, and scleritis in 1.8%.

Sarcoidosis

Twenty-five percent have eye involvement and granulomatous uveitis is the most common finding. It is usually bilateral and more commonly involves the anterior than the posterior uveal tract.

Behçet's Syndrome

This condition is seen more commonly in Mediterranean countries and Japan, but also occurs in this country. It requires three of the following manifestations be present: (1) recurrent aphthous stomatitis, (2) similar ulcerations in the genital area, (3) uveitis, (4) synovitis, (5) cutaneous vasculitis, and (6) meningo-encephalitis. The classic triad has been oral and genital ulcerations and uveitis. Other commonly found features include a history of migratory superficial thrombophlebitis and erythema nodosum. In Japan, Behçet's accounts for 20% of the cases of uveitis.

Relapsing Polychondritis

Eye involvement occurs in the majority of patients and includes iritis, episcleritis, and conjunctivitis.

SUGGESTED READING

1. Pessler HH. The eye in rheumatic disease. Bull Rheum Dis. 1985; 35:1-8.

PART IV.

OVERVIEW OF TREATMENT OF RHEUMATIC DISEASES

Chapter 43

Deciding Whether, and How, to Treat

We have two major goals whenever we see a patient. One is to define the cause for his complaints, that is, diagnose the illness. The other is to provide symptomatic or definitive treatment. Deciding whether or not treatment is indicated and choosing which one to use may be the most difficult decision we make. Three main factors go into this decision—the patient, her specific illness and how she and you see it, and what's known or popular about the various treatment options possible.

THE IDEAL TREATMENT

Ideally, a treatment should be highly efficacious and totally devoid of side effects, affordable, and acceptable to the patient. The patient receiving it should be highly compliant with the treatment regimen and an accurate reporter of any changes in the illness. Furthermore, the data on which clinical efficacy is based should have been obtained in patients with the same illness as your patient, and with the same extent of disease. For example, a treatment that may be efficacious early in the illness in preventing joint loss, such as antibiotics for a septic joint, may not be capable of preserving the joint if started too late in the course of illness. However, it could still be indicated since it may still be capable of modifying an undesirable complication like bacteremia and possible septic death.

Studies done to evaluate the treatment you are contemplating should have looked at the appropriate outcome measures important to your patient and you, and the results obtained should be reliable. The reproducibility and applicability of the results of the study and the safety and efficacy of the treatment must be evaluated by studies free of systemic error (*bias*) and random error (*chance*). Since there is always the possibility that the results are due to chance, some measure of this risk that the results are due to chance is calculated by determining the probability (p) value. The level of this probability that is acceptable to us is then decided. Usually we use p less than 0.05, or 95% or greater likelihood that the result is *not* due to chance. Another way to express and report this probability is the 95% confidence interval, which tells us the range of values within which the results are likely to fall 95% of the time.

In fact, only some of the treatments currently in use for rheumatic diseases have been established as efficacious in case-controlled, randomized, double-blind clinical trials. One of the reasons for this is the relatively low number of patients with a given rheumatic illness seen in any one institution. For this reason, many of the few well designed clinical trials have arisen through the cooperative efforts of investigators at several different medical centers. These researchers have been willing to adhere closely to tightly defined protocols designed with the goal to eliminate all possible sources of bias (or systematic error).

Another source of information regarding treatment comes from "open" studies, so-called because the intervention is known to both the patient and the physician, and the untreated group used as control patients based on historical reminiscence. While this is less than optimal, apparently successful open trials and "n of l" trials are often the impetus to develop better-designed and controlled double-blinded studies in single or multiple institutions. Therapeutic trials in only one patient, "n of l" trials, or case reports may be quite valuable if the measured outcome is objective, easily measured, and well-known, and the treatment is blinded to examiner and examined. The intricacies of design of clinical trials has been the subject of several excellent textbooks and articles, and interested readers are referred to them for further discussion.

MEASURING OUTCOME

Outcome from any illness depends on more than just treatment. In studies of several conditions, several factors have repeatedly appeared as important prognostic indicators. They include:

1. *Level of education* unrelated to socioeconomic status. Perhaps the additional knowledge one acquires through schooling provides a greater sense of understanding and control?
2. *Compliance*, even with ineffective or dangerous therapies. This was demonstrated in the Coronary Drug Project, which looked at treatment of hypercholesterolemia with clofibrate. Despite the adverse outcome associated with clofibrate, patients that were compliant with placebo had a much better prognosis than non-compliant patients from either group. Whether this phenomenon is due to some positive effect from following recommendations made by trusted professionals or whether it actually identifies a subgroup of individuals with a better inherent chance of improving due to their personality and faith in treatment is unclear.
3. *Placebo* effect. This effect has been known for decades although several misconceptions about it are widely held. Patients with "real" disease are *more* likely to respond to it than patients with psychoneurosis. The affected population in any given study runs about 40% but may range from 10-80% as shown in some of the multicenter studies on H_2 blockers for peptic ulcer disease. Some physicians are more "placebogenic" than others (not a bad attribute to have if you want to help your patients to feel better). The dose, route of administration, and physical characteristics of the placebo (like color, taste, etc.) also influence its efficacy. Although usually considered an effect to be avoided in therapeutic trials, in clinical practice it is a useful confounder in improving outcome in your patients.

RECOMMENDED GUIDELINES FOR TREATMENT

1. *Decide why you should treat.* The reasons may vary, but in general, should be dictated by the morbidity and likely outcome of untreated disease, and patient's wishes and ability to comply with the treatment, the available evidence that the treatment works in similar patients, and the potential toxicity of the treatment in general and in your patient in particular. Treating to make us, the physicians, feel better, is *very* rarely (if ever) indicated, unless we are the ones who are ill, in which cases we should be the ones that take the treatment.
2. *Decide how you will monitor whether or not the treatment is working.* Ideally, you should be able to identify both subjective and objective

measures of improvement, e.g., well-being and serum complement levels.

3. *Learn about the drug* you are planning to use and how and when you will monitor for potential drug toxicity. Indications, efficacy, possible and predictable side effects, pharmacology, necessary dose adjustment in patients with renal or hepatic dysfunction, drug interactions, and recommended monitoring for drug toxicity.
4. *Share with the patient the reasons you want to treat,* how you will follow progress against the illness, why you think it should work, what you know about the drug, and what the possible risks are. In summary, *teach your patient.*
5. *Give written, easily readable instructions* on how to take the medication(s) and when and where to call or go if anything goes wrong.
6. *At each return visit,* ask the patient what prescribed and over-the-counter preparations he is taking and in what dose and frequency, and make a notation of it in the medical record.
7. If your patient is not improving despite your best efforts, *send her for a second opinion* to a recognized expert. Never chastise or feel personally attacked if a patient doing poorly wishes other opinions. The result will be either support for your approach or an increase in your knowledge.

GLOSSARY OF ADDITIONAL TERMS USED IN EVALUATING CLINICAL TRIALS

Type I error: Same as the alpha error, it is measured by the p value. It is the probability that a favorable treatment outcome is due to chance rather than a true difference.

Type II error: Same as the beta error or the "power" of the study to detect a true difference. It is the probability that a negative finding is wrong and that the treatment in fact works, but your study did not have a sufficient number of patients or a great enough measure of improvement to show efficacy.

Meta-analysis: a process of re-analyzing results of several similar intervention studies by combining the populations studied and their outcome. May be quite useful when strict guidelines are used in "lumping" populations from different studies.

Regression to the mean: The statistical tendency for extreme values in a distribution to have lower values with repeat measurements.

Hawthorne effect: The tendency for individuals participating in a study to improve just from the attention being provided to them rather than from the intervention itself.

Bonferoni correction: A method to approximate a more acceptable p value in studies involving multiple comparisons, since each comparison has a one in 20 (0.05) chance of being spuriously found significant. It is done by dividing the desired level of significance for the experiment as a whole (usually 0.05%) by the number of comparisons being made between the treated population and the control group.

For example, if you are looking at 10 paired comparisons, the alpha level of significance 0.05 is divided by the number of paired comparisons (10). Therefore, for the particular study with 10 comparisons, a more reasonable alpha level would be a p of 0.005 or less.

SUGGESTED READINGS

1. Fletcher RH, Fletcher SW, Wagner EH. *Clinical Epidemiology, the Essentials*. Second edition. Baltimore: Williams and Wilkins, 1988.

2. Hennekens CH, Buring JE. *Epidemiology in Medicine*. Boston: Little, Brown, and Company, 1987.

Chapter 44

Nonsteroidal Anti-inflammatory Drugs and Other Analgesics

Nonsteroidal anti-inflammatory drugs (NSAIDs) are frequently used as "first line" agents in the treatment of minor to severe inflammation. These inflammatory conditions include most forms of arthritis, bursitis, tendonitis, as well as acute over-use syndromes. Many NSAIDs are currently available (see Table 1) and it is important to keep the following in mind:

—the NSAIDs have minimal differences in effectiveness, and all are similar to aspirin in full anti-inflammatory dose;
—all NSAIDs have comparable risk of side effects, and all are safer than aspirin;
—all NSAIDs should be administered with meals;
—none affect the underlying disease process or hasten healing;
—all NSAIDs work for all types of inflammation; and
—all are fair analgesics at low dose and anti-inflammatory only at higher doses; anti-inflammatory action is maintained only with regular, daily use.

General Principles in Choosing a NSAID

Despite the fact that all NSAIDs have identifical proposed mechanisms of action and similar overall efficacy, it is a well-recognized phenomenon that the individual patient may respond well to one NSAID and not to another or have significant toxicity on one but not on another. It is useful to know the general chemical groupings of these agents (Table

44.1). If a patient derives no benefit or has significant side effects with one NSAID, a replacement NSAID is generally chosen from a different class of NSAID. (However, even within a given class, an individual's response to each agent may differ greatly.)

Other general principles need to be considered in the selection and optimal use of NSAIDS.

—The cost of NSAIDs variest greatly. Aspirin is the least expensive, but its toxicities can be expensive.
—Adequate trials (in rheumatoid arthritis) of 3-4 weeks for each NSAID used are recommended.
—Compliance varies with dosing schedule as well as toxicity profile. Medications taken on a q.d. basis (e.g., piroxicam or slow-release indomethacin) are better received than drugs requiring

Table 44.1.
Classes of NSAIDS

Salicylates	*Propionic Acids*	*Acetic Acids*	*Phenylacetic Acids*
Aspirin-regular or enteric-coated (Ecotrin)	Ibuprofen (Motrin, Rufen,) Advil, Nuprin)	Indomethacin (Indocin, Indocin SR)	Diclofenac (Voltaren)
Choline magnesium (Trilisate)	Naproxen (Naprosyn)	Sulindac (Clinoril)	
Salsalate (Disalcid)	Fenoprofen (Nalfon)	Tolmetin (Tolectin)	
Diflunisal (Dolobid)	Ketoprofen (Orudis)		
Magnesium salicylate (Magan)	Flurbiprofen (Ansaid)		

Fenamates	*Oxicams*	*Pyrazoles*
Meclofenamate (Meclomen)	Piroxicam (Feldene)	Phenylbutazone (Butazolidin)

t.i.d. or q.i.d. dosing (e.g., aspirin, ibuprofen, tolmetin, or regular indomethacin), however the longer half-life increases toxicity.
—Maximum efficacy might not be reached until maximum recommended doses are used.
—Multiple NSAIDs taken together generally have no added benefit but always enhance toxicity.
—Recent reports of NSAID-related deaths in the *elderly* demonstrate the need for caution when treating this population.

COMMON SIDE EFFECTS ON NSAIDS

A. Central Nervous System
   1. Headaches, altered mentation , or altered consciousness may be encountered with any of the NSAIDs. Most commonly seen with
      —indomethacin
      —phenylbutazone
      —high dose aspirin (the elderly may develop CNS changes despite subtherapeutic levels of salicylate).

B. Gastrointestinal
   1. Gastritis, gastric ulcers, and esophagitis have been observed with all NSAIDs. They are most commonly seen with aspirin and indomethacin.
   2. Active gastric or duodenal disease should be treated with H_2 blockers and/or sucralfate plus discontinuing the NSAID. Misoprostol, a prostaglandin analogue, is a newer cytoprotective agent, approved for prophylaxis of gastric ulceration in high risk patients. A dose of 100 μg q.i.d. is usually effective.
   3. If the NSAID cannot be stopped, healing of ulcers with optimal therapy will be delayed.
   4. Diarrhea is possible with any NSAID but most commonly observed with meclofenamate.

C. Platelet Inhibition
   1. Aspirin irreversibly inhibits platelet aggregation. This platelet dysfunction persists until newly synthesized (non-acetylated) platelets can replace those exposed to aspirin. This takes 10 to 12 days.
   2. NSAID inhibition of platelet aggregation is reversible and therefore related to the drug's half-life.

3. Aspirin and NSAIDs should be stopped prior to surgery to minimize bleeding problems.
   —aspirin stopped two weeks pre-op;
   —tolmetin and the propionic acid derivatives stopped 24 hours pre-op;
   —naproxen, indomethacin, and sulindac stopped 48 hours pre-op;
   —piroxicam stopped 72 or more hours pre-op.

D. Renal Toxicity
   1. Decreased GFR occurs with all NSAIDs. With shorter-activating agents (ibuprofen or tolmetin) or sulindac, this effect is minimized.
   2. Sodium retention is observed with all NSAIDs but especially indomethacin and phenylbutazone. Care must be taken in patients with heart disease.
   3. Patients on potassium-retaining diuretics (Dyazide or Aldactazide) may develop life-threatening hyperkalemia on NSAIDs, secondary to hyporeninemic hypoaldosteronism.
   4. Idiosyncratic interstitial nephritis occurs rarely with NSAIDs. It is characterized by sudden, reversible renal shutdown and eosinophiluria.

LESS COMMON SIDE EFFECTS OF NSAIDS

1. changes in visual acuity
2. aseptic meningitis (primarily from ibuprofen)
3. granulomatous hepatitis and acute pancreatitis (with sulindac)
4. bronchospasm, urticaria, anaphylaxis
5. hypersensitivity pneumonitis
6. cytopenias of varying degrees up to aplastic anemia.

Any unexplained new illness in a patient on a NSAID should suggest to you a possible adverse drugged effect from it. Discontinuation and observation while further evaluating the patient is your safest course of action.

NSAID INTERACTIONS WITH OTHER DRUGS

Antihypertensives (beta blockers, thiazides, and captopril)
—the blood pressure-lowering effects ar reduced by all NSAIDs except for sulindac.

Potassium-sparing diuretics (Dyazide, Aldactazide, and Maxide)
—acute renal failure and life-threatening hyperkalemia may develop with any NSAID

Antiglaucoma agents (Diamox, Daranide, and Neptazane)
—metabolic acidosis may develop with any NSAID

Coumadin (warfarin) and sulfonylureas
—NSAIDs cause protein-binding displacement leading to prolonged anti-coagulation or hypoglycemia.

Corticosteroids
—aspirin clearance is increased

Lithium, methotrexate, and chlorpropamide
—aspirin increases renal tubular secretion of these compounds.

ANALGESICS USE IN RHEUMATIC DISEASE

As mentioned in the preceding section, NSAIDs have analgesic properties in addition to their anti-inflammatory activities. Frequently, the pain relief afforded by NSAIDs alone is not satisfactory and other therapeutic approaches are necessary. In some inflammatory processes, like rheumatoid arthritis and psoriatic arthritis, there are "second line" agents to turn to that may have greater efficacy (and greater toxicity). In other forms of arthritis, like osteoarthritis and CPPD disease, there are no specific "second line" options. In either case, the analgesic regimen should be optimized prior to proceeding on to more toxic agents.

General Approach

If adequate trials of NSAIDs have proved insufficient in reducing pain, *acetaminophen* in regularly administered doses should be added. A suggested starting dose of acetaminophen is 650 mg taken three or four times per day, in patients without substantial liver disease. Other analgesics such as propoxyphene (Darvon), pentazocine (Talwin), or codeine have not been superior to acetaminophen in relieving arthritis pain, and, since they are addictive, have no role in treating chronic pain problems. If the combination of acetaminophen and a NSAID does not result in adequate symptomatic relief, the "first line" approach to musculoskeletal pain treatment is completed by the addition of a tricyclic antidepressant. In addition to their sedative and antidepressant activities, tricyclics (amitriptyline and doxepin) have direct central analgesic effects and may potentiate other forms of analgesics.

It is important to remember that approaching pain management by a purely pharmacologic means is doomed to failure. Pain—especially chronic pain in musculoskeletal disorders—is a complex process that requires attention to other factors. Psychological and social components need to be explored. The total analgesic program should also include scheduled rest, exercise, and relaxation programs. Patient education and the use of physical medicine modalities are also important.

Should narcotic analgesics ever be used for joint disease?

In long-standing arthritis, joint destruction may progress to where pain is *mechanical* ("bone on bone") rather than *inflammatory*. In this setting of end-stage joint disease, simple analgesics may be more effective and less toxic than NSAIDs or second line agents. Narcotic analgesics might be justified after a long and adequate trial with non-narcotic analgesics, and specifically when:

—surgery is anticipated in the near future, and in the very immediate postoperative period

—or where the risk of narcotic addiction is offset by the improved quality of life.

SUGGESTED READINGS

1. Simon LS, Mills JA. Nonsteroidal anti-inflammatory drugs. N. Engl J Med. 1980; 302:1179-1185, 1237-1243.

2. Schlegel SI, Paulus HE. Update on NSAID use in rheumatic diseases. Bull Rheum Dis. 1986, 36: 1-8.

3. Csuka ME, McCarty DJ. Aspirin and the treatment of rheumatoid arthritis. Rheum Clin North Am. 1989; 15:439-54.

4. Roth SH. Merits and liability of NSAID therapy. Rheum Clin North Am. 1989; 15: 479-98.

5. Barrier, CH, Hirschowitz BI. Controversies in the detection and management of non steroidal anti-inflammatory drug-induced side effects of the upper gastrointestinal tract. Arthritis Rheum. 1989; 32:926-932.

Chapter 45

Second Line Agents in Rheumatoid Arthritis (Slow Acting and Cytotoxic Drugs)

Second line drugs, previously known as slow-acting drugs, have been used in the treatment of rheumatoid arthritis for several decades. They are administered when patients are considered to have failed basic therapy with salicylates or non-steroidal anti-inflammatory drugs and physical and occupational therapy. The decision to use these drugs is based on clinical activity and functional and anatomic class. (See Chapter 26.) Common characteristics of these drugs are: (1) slow onset of action, (2) suppression of disease activity that may last for months or years with continued administration of the drug, (3) quiescent inflammation for weeks or months after the drug(s) has been discontinued, (4) possible tissue protective effects, and (5) minimal anti-inflammatory effects (although cytotoxic agents probably have primarily anti-inflammatory effects). The choice of drugs among this class is usually from the safest (anti-malarials) to the most toxic (e.g., D-penicillamine). Commonly, patients with RA will eventually be tried on 3–5 of these drugs.

I. Slow-Acting Drugs

1. Antimalarial Drugs

   Antimalarial drugs such as hydroxychloroquine (Plaquenil) or chloroquine (Aralen) are prescribed for patients with inflammatory arthritides including progressive, erosive rheumatoid arthritis, systemic lupus erythematosus, and juvenile chronic arthritis. They have limited utility in patients with psoriatic arthritis and questionable benefit in the treatment of patients with peripheral arthritis associated with the spondyloarthropathies.

Dosages and onset of action

These drugs are rapidly absorbed and quickly cleared from the plasma. Although levels plateau in the plasma and urine in 2 to 5 weeks, the drug continues to accumulate in liver, spleen, kidneys, skin, and leukocytes. It is tightly bound to pigmented tissue such as is present in the eye where macular toxicity can develop. Efficacy from antimalarial therapy is rarely seen before six weeks and is more likely to occur between four to six months after beginning treatment. The usual dose is 5-7 mg/kg of body weight per day, and the daily dose of hydroxychloroquine should not exceed 400 mg. The drug is administered as a 200-mg scored tablet.

Side Effects

Although these drugs have many reported toxicities, they are usually well tolerated. They only rarely cause reversible bone marrow suppression so monitoring with frequent blood counts is not necessary. The most serious complication from these drugs is macular pigmentation. This can progress to visual loss if the patient is not monitored with ophthalmologic evaluations every six months, checking peripheral vision to red and white light. Any loss of red light peripheral vision is interpreted as possible-pre-maculopathy and is an indication for discontinuation of the drug. The abnormality then reverses very quickly. Hydroxychloroquine is felt to be less toxic to the eye than chloroquine and should be the drug of choice among antimalarials. It is felt that the risk for eye damage correlates with exceeding the recommended daily dose rather than the total cumulative dose. A characteristic "bull's eye" retina lesion has been described.

Other common toxicities include gastrointestinal intolerance such as cramps, abdominal distention, nausea, and diarrhea. Cutaneous side effects such as rash, and changes in pigmentation of hair and skin are sometimes seen. Rarely, there are neurologic side effect such as tinnitus, vertigo, vestibular dysfunction, and headaches. Myopathy and cardiomyopathy are very rare but serious side effects which have recognizable pathologic findings on biopsy. Prompt discontinuation of the drug is indicated for this toxicity which is usually rapidly reversible.

2. Gold

Gold is considered by some rheumatologists to be the best drug available to modify the course of rheumatoid arthritis. It, like antimalarials and penicillamine, belongs to a class of slow-acting drugs which require saturation of tissues (4 to 6 months) before a therapeutic benefit can occur. It is indicated in the treatment of progressive, erosive rheumatoid arthritis and is used less frequently in other inflammatory arthropathies such as psoriatic arthritis and juvenile chronic arthritis. It is not indicated for mild rheumatoid disease until adequate trials of nonsteroidal anti-inflammatory drugs are given without adequately controlling the disease.

There are presently three preparations of gold available in the United States, two parenteral forms: gold thioglucose (Solganal) and gold thiomaleate (Myochrysine) and an oral preparation, auranofin (Ridaura). Auranofin is thought to have a slight earlier onset of action and less severe toxicity (renal and hematopoetic) than parenteral gold, but may be less effective that the intramuscular preparations.

Dosages and onset of action

Auranofin is administered as a 3-mg tablet given twice daily. The dose can be increased to 9 mg/day to gain additional therapeutic benefit. The parenteral forms are given in 25- to 50-mg doses weekly to achieve a cumulative dose of 500 mg to 1 gm (20 weeks), after which the frequency of injection is decreased to alternate weeks for several months. Eventually, the injections can be given at monthly intervals for maintenance. Usually a test dose of 10 mg is given the first week to check for severe toxicity before administering the 25- to 50-mg weekly dose. Doses can be modified according to toxicity, but the drug must be continued for at least 4 to 6 months before one can see therapeutic benefit. In fact, there may be responses occurring as late as 9 to 12 months after therapy is started.

Side Effects

Although gold compounds were considered the backbone of therapy for progressive rheumatoid arthritis, considerable concern must be exercised during their administration because of potential toxicity. Only physicians experienced in using gold and treating its serious toxicities should be prescribing it. Gold toxicity can be divided into mild and severe reactions. Mild toxicities include: stomatitis, pruritus, local rash, and a metallic taste. In addition, with Myochrysine, one can also see a vasomotor reaction soon after parenteral administration, causing dizziness, flushing and syncope, and (rarely) associated myocardial infarction. This is referred to as a "nitritoid" reaction. More serious toxicities include bone marrow suppression, causing thrombocytopenia, leukopenia, or aplastic anemia; membranous glomerulonephritis causing proteinuria and nephrotic syndrome; and exfoliative dermatitis. Other serious but rare toxicities are enterocolitis, cholestatic jaundice, and "gold pneumonitis." Diarrhea is common 15 to 20% in patients taking auranofin, worse with doses above 6 mg q.d.

Because of the potential for bone marrow suppression and nephropathy, initial weekly complete blood counts with differential (CBC), platelet counts, and urinalysis must be done. White blood counts should not fall below 3500 nor platelet count below 150,000/mm^3. In addition to watching for the absolute values, rapid falls in counts (i.e., platelet counts falling by 100,000 or white count by 2-5,000) should arouse suspicions of impending serious toxicity. Gold therapy should be stopped until the values are repeated and found to be satisfactory. A flow chart is recommended to follow patterns of change of platelet and white blood cell counts. Prior to administering the weekly injection, patients should be asked about and examined for stomatitis and pruritic rash. Gold can be administered in maintenance doses for many years without significant cumulative side effects. In fact, most serious toxicity to gold occurs within the first 6 to 12 months of therapy.

3. D-Penicillamine

Penicillamine, a product of metabolism of penicillin, is a slow-acting drug used to treat active RA and juvenile chronic arthritis. Penicillin allergy is not a contraindication to treatment. It is more toxic than other slow-acting and cytotoxic drugs and as such should not be used prior to trials of these drugs. Many studies have reported it to be as effective as gold salts.

Dosage and onset of action

It is administered either in tablet or capsule form, and the dose is slowly increased from 250 mg/d to 750 mg/d, the "go low, go slow," method. It takes 4 to 6 months to get a response from the drug. Rapid increase in daily dose (more frequent than 250 mg/month) is associated with increased risk of toxicity.

Side Effects

The drug is contraindicated in unreliable patients who will not come for regular blood and urine testing. Side effects of penicillamine such as bone marrow suppression and nephropathy are comparable to gold, except that risk for thrombocytopenia from penicillamine is higher than for gold and can occur at any time while the patient is on the drug. The CBC, platelet count, and urinalyses should be monitored the same as recommended for gold therapy. Patients should be monitored weekly initially, and, once a steady daily dose is reached, patients should be monitored every 2-4 weeks.

Hypogeusia occurs commonly up to three months after starting the drug and usually clears despite continuation of the drug. Uncommon severe toxicities unique to penicillamine are immunologically mediated diseases such as myasthenia gravis, dermato/polymyositis, Goodpasture's syndrome, pemphigus, lupus erythematosus, and Sjögren's syndrome. These diseases subside upon withdrawal of the drug but may require therapy for some time afterwards. This drug should be administered only by a rheumatologist or someone very familiar with its toxicities.

4. Sulfasalazine

This drug was originally designed specifically for treatment of rheumatoid arthritis. It consists of one molecule of salicylic acid linked by an azo bond to one molecule of the sulfonamide sulfapyridine. Early studies in the late 1940s showed favorable results, but one negative study was reported around the time that steroids were first introduced and thought to cure RA. Sulfasalazine (SSZ) became the treatment of choice in ulcerative colitis, but was not re-discovered as a second line agent for RA until this decade.

Dosage and onset of action

SSZ is not yet FDA-approved for treatment of RA but is being used with increasing frequency by rheumatologists because of its relatively early onset of action (about 6-8 weeks from the time full dose of 2-3 gm q.d. begins) and ease of administration. The enteric-coated tablets of 500 mg each are best tolerated, and dosing starts with 500 mg b.i.d. for 1-2 weeks. The dose is then increased to 1 gm b.i.d., and, if necessary, to 1.5 gm b.i.d. In most trials, a favorable response has occurred in 60-75% of patients. A known previous adverse reaction to sulfa drugs and/or salicylates is a contraindication to its use.

Side Effects

Most side effects occur within the first 3 months of therapy. GI intolerance and musculocutaneous toxicity are usually mild and respond to discontinuing the drug. However, more serious and potentially fatal skin reactions can rarely occur. Leukopenia, agranulocytosis, aplastic anemia, thrombocytopenia, hemolytic anemia, megaloblastic anemia, methemoglobinemia, and sulfhemoglobinemia have all been reported. The incidence is probably less than 1-2% and, with few exceptions, reversible. There have been a few reported fatalities. Other reported adverse effects include a lupus-like syndrome, CNS symptoms, and occasional allergic interstitial pneumonitis. A dose-dependent toxic hepatitis may also occur.

Toxicity monitoring includes patient education, so any unusual or new symptoms are reported, and CBC with differential, platelet count, and chemistry profile should be done every three weeks for three months. Every 6-8 weeks thereafter is sufficient once a stable dose is reached.

II. Cytotoxic Drugs

1. Methotrexate

Methotrexate is a folic acid antagonist that has recently been widely used for the treatment of rheumatoid arthritis. Its efficacy was first recognized in the treatment of psoriatic arthritis. Subsequently, it was tried in patients with RA. It provides significant and anti-inflammatory effect although it is not a nonsteroidal anti-inflammatory drug.

Dosage and onset of action

Its onset of action begins in 4-6 weeks after therapy is started. The disease usually flares 3-4 weeks after it is discontinued. The drug can be conveniently taken only one day per week, and the dose can range from 5 mg-15 mg weekly, depending upon efficacy and toxicity. The drug is available as a 2.5-mg tablet. It can also be given parenterally although there is no demonstrable advantage for giving the drug that way.

Side Effects

Most side effects of methotrexate are dose related, reflecting the effect of the drug on normal, rapidly proliferating tissues, and are more frequent in people with decreased renal function. Mild toxicity includes stomatitis, nausea, vomiting, and diarrhea. Bone marrow suppression can occur but is usually reversible and can be regulated by lowering the dose of the drug. The drop in blood counts is rarely as precipitous as they can be with gold and penicillamine.

Unpredictable but serious side effects are development of pulmonary and liver inflammation and fibrosis. Pulmonary symptoms such as cough, fever and progressive dyspnea can occur either acutely or chronically and are an indication for prompt discontinuation of the drug. Lung involvement may occur very early in therapy. Liver damage may be minimized by weekly "pulse" administration of the drug instead of divided doses and by avoiding treatment of patients with certain risk factors such as renal insufficiency, alcoholism, obesity, and diabetes mellitus.

Although patients receiving methotrexate should be monitored by monthly blood counts and liver function tests, it is recognized that these values may not correlate with serious liver damage or the development of fibrosis. The risk for cirrhosis appears low, so at present the recommendation that patients receiving methotrexate have liver biopsies performed after a total cumulative dose of 1.5 gm or after three years of therapy is not being made as strongly as earlier.

2. Azathioprine

Azathioprine is a purine analog antimetabolite which has FDA approval for use in rheumatoid arthritis. It is also used extensively in lupus nephritis and steroid-resistant polymyositis/dermatomyositis. It is probably one of the safest cytotoxic drugs available and has long been used in the treatment of kidney transplant patients.

Dosage and onset of action

It is generally given at doses of 1-2.5 mg/kg body weight per day and it takes 2-3 months to see therapeutic benefit after beginning therapy.

Side Effects

Long-term studies suggest that 15% of patients receiving the drug may discontinue it because of toxicity. The two major toxic effects are gastrointestinal and bone marrow suppression. Gastrointestinal complaints (which occur in up to 19% of patients) include nausea, vomiting, and, less commonly, ulceration and diarrhea. Rare cases of "idiosyncratic" pancreatitis and hepatitis are reported.

Hematologic toxicity usually manifests itself as leukopenia (sometimes neutropenia). For this reason, CBC and platelet counts should be obtained initially weekly, and, once a stable dose is reached, once monthly. White counts should not fall below 2500 and platelets below 150,000. The risk for infection is increased in patients receiving azathioprine. Both common microbes or those seen in immunocompromised hosts such as *Pneumocystis carinii* may be involved even in the absence of severe leukopenia.

The most important long-term risk for this drug is the potential for development of malignancies, especially non-Hodgkin's lymphomas and leukemia. This side effect was first recognized in renal transplant patients who had a 10% incidence of lymphoreticular malignancy. Several reports of patients with RA developing similar malignancies have appeared. The overall risk is low and considerably less than in renal transplant patients.

3. Cyclophosphamide

There was initial enthusiasm in the early 1970s about clinical trials of cyclophosphamide, an alkylating agent, in rheumatoid arthritis. Several double blind studies of 8-9 months' duration showed significant improvement of many criteria of disease activity.

Dosage and onset of action

The average daily dose employed is 1.8-2 mg/kg body weight, although some advocate starting with 25 mg q.d. and increasing by 25 mg daily every 1-2 months while monitoring the cell counts for cytopenias.

Side Effects

Despite the obvious clinical improvement, serious toxicities were noted which significantly limit the long-term usefulness of the drug. The early side effects include stomatitis, alopecia, dysuria, hemorrhagic cystitis, and herpes zoster. Far more serious, however, is the late toxicity of malignancy including lymphoproliferative disorders, solid tumors, and bladder cancer. The risk for bladder carcinoma seems to be directly related to the total cumulative cyclophosphamide dose received. Because the risk for serious toxicity seems to outweigh the benefits in patients with uncomplicated RA, it is now recommended that this drug not be used if others are available. The exception is for rheumatoid vasculitis where the combination of prednisone and cyclophophamide may be life-saving.

SUGGESTED READINGS

1. Maksymowych W, Russell AS. Antimalarials in rheumatology: Efficacy and safety. Sem Arthritis Rheum. 1987; 16:206-21.

2. Drugs for rheumatoid arthritis. Med Lett Drugs Therapeutics. 1987; 29:21-24.

3. Pinals RS. Sulfasalazine in rheumatic disease. Sem Arthritis Rheum. 1988; 17;246-59.

Chapter 46

Steroids in Rheumatic Diseases

Glucocorticoids are 21-carbon steroid molecules whose major activity is dependent upon the presence of a hydroxyl group at the C_{11} site of the molecule. Cortisol, normally produced by the adrenal cortex, is under direct control of ACTH produced by the anterior pituitary gland and under indirect control of the hypothalamus. ACTH stimulates production of cortisol which, in turn, provides negative feedback either at the level of the pituitary gland or the hypothalamus or both. Prednisone and cortisone, two of the most commonly used steroid drugs, have keto groups at the C_{11} site and require transformation to the hydroxyl compounds, prednisolone, and cortisol respectively, to produce maximal physiological effects. This C_{11} hydroxylation step occurs in the liver, and while most patients can metabolize these oral compounds to the active form, patients with liver disease or with a faulty hydroxylation system will appear unresponsive to these drugs. In these patients, active drugs are preferred (e.g., prednisolone or methyl prednisolone).

Glucocorticoids are widely used in the treatment of many rheumatic diseases such as systemic lupus erythematosus, rheumatoid arthritis, inflammatory muscle diseases, Sjögren's syndrome, and the vasculitides, including polyarteritis nodosa, temporal (giant cell) arteries, allergic granulomatosis, and hypersensitivity vasculitis.

DOSAGES AND PREPARATIONS

There are many forms of corticosteroids available. These range from oral and parenteral forms to topical preparations. (See Chapter 6.)

1. *Oral Preparations*: These drugs are well absorbed from the gastrointestinal tract and are 90% protein bound.

Oral Glucocorticoid Preparation	Anti-Inflammatory Potency	Equivalent Dose (mg)
Hydrocortisone	1	20
*Cortisone	0.8	25
*Prednisone	4	5
Prednisolone	4	5
Methylprednisolone	5	4
Dexamethasone	30	0.75

*inactive until metabolized to C_{11} hydroxy form.

Dosages Available:
Prednisone: 1-, 2.5-, 5-, 10-, 20-, and 50-mg tablets.
Prednisolone: 1-, 2.5-, and 5-mg tablets.
Methylprednisolone: 2-, 4-, 8-, 16-, 24-, 32-mg tablets.
Dexamethasone:: 0.25-, 0.5-, 0.75-, 1.5-, 4-, and 6-mg tablets.

2. *Parenteral Preparations*
These drugs, given intra-articularly or at periarticular sites of local inflammation, can be very effective in relieving pain, swelling, and warmth. The duration of response varies from several days to months (see Chapter 6). Large doses of steroids injected into large joints may be absorbed and suppress the plasma cortisol level but to a lesser extent than chronic oral or parenteral doses. The parenteral preparations available are listed below.
Methyl prednisolone vial: 40, 125, 500, 1000 mg/ml
Dexamethasone: 4 mg/ml in 1-, 5-, 25-ml vial, or 24 mg/ml in 5-and 10-ml containers
Parenteral administration is reserved primarily for two groups of patients:
a. The acutely and severely ill patient with a rapidly progressive vasculitis or lupus nephritis, in whom 1000-mg "boluses" are given daily for 1-3 days to achieve as quick a control over the inflammatory process as possible, followed by 1 mg/kg daily oral or parenteral dose plus a cytotoxic dose when indicated. Some rheumatologists prefer to give the same "mega dose" of 1000-mg in four equal parenteral doses distributed over 24 hours to increase even more the anti-inflammatory effect.

b. The rheumatoid arthritis patient with active polyarticular synovitis who either has not yet received adequate cumulative doses of a slow-acting/remission inducing agent or who appears to be failing on these drugs. Either an occasional intravenous bolus of 1000 mg or intermittent intramuscular administration of 1 mg/kg have been used. While some rheumatologist prefer these approaches, others prefer small (less than 10 mg) daily or alternate day oral doses, which have established a longer record of safety.

MECHANISMS OF ACTION

Glucocorticoids are used in treatment of rheumatic diseases for their anti-inflammatory and immunosuppressive effects. The mechanisms by which these drugs produce such effects are exceedingly complex. Steroids can cause leukocyte movement with redistributes cells and can result in lymphopenia, monocytopenia and eosinopenia and polymorphonuclear leukocytosis. In addition to effects on the apparent number of cellular elements in the blood, steroids also affect the function of many cells. Lymphocyte activities, such as delayed hypersensitivity, proliferation in response to antigens, and regulatory effects on helper and suppressor cell populations, are suppressed. Monocyte/macrophage activities, including bactericidal activity, blockage of Fc receptor binding and function are also suppressed. When steroids are used in very high doses—suprapharmacologic doses, neutrophil chemotaxis is inhibited as well. Finally, steroids inhibit phospholipase A2 which releases arachidonic acid from cell membranes, the first step in the production of inflammatory prostaglandins and leukotrienes.

SIDE EFFECTS AND TOXICITY

Although glucocorticoids can produce dramatic results in acutely ill patients, the side effects of these drugs can be equally as dramatic. As with many other drugs, side effects vary directly with increasing doses of the drug and duration of use. Suppression of the pituitary-adrenal axis for about one week can occur in patients taking 50 mg of prednisone daily for only five days. Since most patients remain on steroids for weeks to years, adrenal suppression can be a serious problem if steroids are inadvertently discontinued or the patient is undergoing excessive stress (e.g., surgery, infection, etc.). In these instances, higher doses of exogenous steroids must be administered to prevent an Addisonian crisis—a withdrawal syndrome characterized by profound nausea, vomiting, malaise, and fever. Postural hypotension and eosinophilia may be noted, but, in general, a high degree of suspicion is your best assistance. These symptoms may occur even with apparently normal levels of plasma cortisol. Alternate day dosing ameliorates symptoms of Cushing's syndrome and allows some recovery of the hypothalamic pituitary-adrenal gland axis but is less efficacious.

Glucocorticoids can affect many organ systems, and few or multiple side effects can be seen in patients. Even chronic low doses of steroids can cause posterior subcapsular cataracts and increased intraocular pressure, hypertension, edema from salt retention, osteoporosis with compression fractures, hyperglycemia, gastritis and ulceration, and severe myopathy. If doses are continued for a long duration or if the patient had prior epidermal atrophy, painless intradermal hemorrhages may occur with minimal trauma. The typical "moon face," buffalo hump, striae, and truncal obesity characteristic of Cushing's syndrome occur from alterations in fat metabolism. Central nervous system effects from steroids are seen in almost all patients, and can be manifested by alterations in mood or be so profound as to cause hallucinations and psychosis when used in high doses. Other severe CNS side effects include depression and seizures.

The most life-threatening complication from steroid use is infection because of the effects of steroids on the immune system. This increased risk exists for bacterial, fungal, and other opportunistic infections in patients who are immunocompromised. Because of the significant risk for toxicity from this highly effective class of drugs, they should be used with caution and for the shortest duration of time deemed to be necessary. If the corticosterids must be continued for more than one month, patients should be closely monitored for gastritis, hypertension, hyperglycemia, glaucoma, cataracts, and osteoporosis. Less common but reported complications include overgrowth of fatty deposits in other areas besides the supraclavicular, bicipital and mid-trunk areas with resultant mass effects. Mediastinal fat increase and myelopathy from epidural fat accumulation are examples.

WORD OF WISDOM

In any patient not improving on prednisone, it is often useful to switch to a similar dose of an active oral steroid like prednisolone or methyl prednisolone and to wait 2-3 weeks before instituting more aggressive therapy.

SUGGESTED READINGS

1. Streck WF, Lockwood DH. Pituitary adrenal recovery following short-term suppression with corticosteroids. Am J Med. 1979; 66:910-914.

2. Liebling MR, Leib E, et al. Pulse methylprednisolone in rheumatoid arthritis. Ann Intern Med. 1981; 94:21-26.

3. Harris ED, Emkey RD, Nichols JE, Newberg A. Low dose prednisone therapy in rheumatoid arthritis: A double-blind study. J Rheumatol 1983; 10:713-17.

4. Masi AT. Low dose glucocorticoid therapy in rheumatoid arthritis: Transitional or selected add-on therapy? J Rheumatol. 1983; 10:675-78.

Chapter 47

Physical Medicine and Rheumatology

Rehabilitative (physical) medicine is an important component in the acute and long-term care of rheumatic disease. By using these non-medicinal modalities, we hope to maximize the patient's function by reducing pain, deformity, and dependence on others.

A. Types of Physical Modalities

1. *Cold Therapy*

   Indications: Cold is important in the treatment of acute sprains, strains, and contusions (see Chapter 20). It reduces pain and increases range of motion in acutely inflamed joints. It also reduces local muscle spasm.

   Contraindications: Cold should not be used in patients with Raynaud's, cryoglobulinemia, impaired circulation, heart failure, or inability to sense or report pain.

   Methods: Ice packs, ice massage, or topical cooling sprays (fluromethane) may be used four to six times daily for 15 to 30 minutes.

2. *Superficial Heat*

   Indications: Superficial heat, like cold, raises the pain threshold of inflamed joints. The local increase in circulation has a paradoxic cooling effect on the joint. This form of heat is also good for minor musculoskeletal pain and in preparation for therapeutic (rehabilitative) exercise.

   Contraindications: Should not be used in patients with impaired sensation, circulation, or cardiovascular function. Recent contusions or hemorrhages, likewise, should not be treated with heat.

Methods: Hot packs (hydrocollator), Hubbard tank, whirlpool, and showers can all raise skin temperature to 43-44°C. Hot paraffin wax and "contrast baths" (alternating hot and cold water baths) are particularly helpful for rheumatoid hands.

3. *Deep Heat (Diathermy)*

   Indications: Deep heat will reduce musculoskeletal pain not associated with inflammatory arthritis. It is also used prior to stretching or range of motion exercises.

   Contraindications: Deep heat will worsen inflammatory arthritis. It should not be used in patients with neuropathies or impaired cardiovascular function. Patients with metal implants, pacemakers, and possible malignancies also should not use diathermy.

   Methods: Microwave—electromagnetic radiation; shortwave—high frequency current, and ultrasound.

4. *Electrical Stimulation*

   Transcutaneous electrical nerve stimulation (TENS) is designed to block peripheral pain perception by selectively stimulating the large cutaneous afferent nerve fibers (blocking nerves in the "gate control" theory of pain). About 50% of patients will report effective pain relief for conditions such as cervical spondylosis, muscle spasm, chest wall syndromes, rheumatoid neuropathy, and radiculopathy associated with disc disease.

5. *Traction*

   Traction is frequently effective in reducing pain associated with disc or bony compression of nerve roots. Cervical traction for 2-20 minutes given two to three times per day is effective if weights are initially started low (five to eight pounds to reduce secondary muscle spasm) and increased gradually to 10-30 pounds. Cervical traction is contraindicated in rheumatoid arthritis with C_1-C_2 instability. Lumbar traction may help relieve back pain or sciatica. Both forms of traction need expert supervision, and their efficacy remains unproven.

6. *Other Modalities*

   Massage is a time-honored approach to the relief of muscle pain, stiffness, and spasm. Therapeutically, it is used prior to stretching or strengthening exercises. No long-term benefit from massage has been documented. *Manipulation*, or forcing a joint beyond its normal range of movement, may result in subjective improvement of musculoskeletal symptoms in patients with non-inflammatory disease. Spinal manipulation, as practiced by chiropractors, has not been shown to be of any long-term benefit although many patients will describe immediate or temporary symptomatic improvement. *Biofeedback* uses myoelectric or Doppler monitoring to permit conscious control of physiologic states such as muscle tension and spasm or Raynaud's phenomenon.

B. Therapeutic Exercises

Therapeutic exercise is a specific program of joint movement to improve musculoskeletal function, to correct musculotendinous impairment, or to enhance well-being. The exercises may be *active* (joint movement provided by patient's own muscles), *passive* (joint movement provided by external source), or *assisted* (a combination of active and passive). The type of exercise prescription will depend on the treatment goal, the patient's functional capacity, and the presence of deformity, effusion, or inflammation in the joint.

1. *Range of motion (ROM) exercises*

   —designed to put a joint through its *full* ROM to prevent contractures and improve joint mobility.

2. *Strengthening exercises*

   —Programs are individually designed to improve muscle strength and bulk following disuse or immobility. Resistive isotonic exercises are contraindicated when joints are inflamed or unstable. *Isometric* exercises involve muscle contraction without joint movement. With *isotonic* exercises, muscle contractions move the joints. *Isokinetic* exercise is a form of isotonic exercise which maintains a constant speed of motion independent of the force applied to a specially designed apparatus.

3. *Relaxation exercises*

   —A program which alternates contraction and relaxation of selected muscle groups can occasionally be helpful in treating muscle stress.

C. Assistive Devices

When pain, limited joint mobility and loss of strength have significantly restricted a patient's activities of daily living (ADLs), a variety of devices are available to improve independence and safety.

1. *Mobility Aids:*

   —Canes, crutches, and walkers are used to "unweight" a diseased weight-bearing joint. Canes and crutches are used on the side opposite the symptomatic joint. Special grips and platform extensions will minimize secondary trauma to the upper extremities using such devices.

2. *Household Aids:*

—Many modifications of a patient's living environment can greatly enhance independence. Patients with pelvic girdle and knee disease are greatly assisted by elevating toilet seats and chairs and special bathtub modifications. Adaptive devices for hairbrushes, toothbrushes, and eating utensils are important to patients with shoulder, elbow, or hand disease. Occupational therapy should be routinely consulted by patients with functional limitations.

D. Orthotic Devices

Orthotics are a group of devices that protect a diseased joint by support or immobilization. Examples of commonly prescribed orthotics are:

1. Lumbosacral orthotic braces are helpful in acute back pain but may hasten osteoporosis and laxity of support muscles.
2. Cervical collars—soft collars are adequate for most cervical impingement problems. The less well-tolerated Philadelphia collar is used in recalcitrant cases. Neurologic deficit or C_1-C_2 instability requires neurosurgical consultation.
3. Wrist and finger splints
4. Knee braces (hinged, Swedish cage, or Lenox-Hill)
5. Metatarsal bars or pads
6. Heel cups for calcaneal spurs
7. Wide toe-box shoes

SUGGESTED READINGS

1. Lehmann JF, Warren CG, Seham SM. Therapeutic heat and cold. Clin Orthop. 1974; 99:207-18.

2. Hicks JE, Nicholas JJ, Swezey RL. *Handbook of Rehabilitative Rheumatology.* Atlanta. Am Rheum Assoc. 1988.

3. Gerber NL, Hicks JE. Rehabilitation in the management of patients with osteoarthritis, in Moskowitz (ed.) *Osteoarthritis.* Philadelphia: W.B. Saunders, 1984.

Chapter 48

Diet

The composition of the diet is important in the function of musculoskeletal and immune systems. For example, a diet deficient in vitamin C can produce scurvy and one deficient in vitamin D, rickets. Excessive dietary amounts of vitamins A or D are also well known to be accompanied by many musculoskeletal changes and symptoms. Zinc deficiency, vitamin A deficiency, and pyridoxine (B6) deficiency have devastating effects on the immune response. At this time, however, the great majority (some would say all) of the currently identified rheumatic diseases and syndromes do not appear due to too much or too little of any one essential or non-essential nutrient or contaminant. Likewise, although the effect of diet composition, particularly fatty acids, has been shown to have an impressive impact on morbidity and mortality of some animal models of rheumatic diseases (like the murine models of SLE), attempts to reproduce these findings in human clinical studies have been few and unimpressive.

It is fairly well accepted that the fatty acid composition of the diet may influence the inflammatory response. Reported studies of diet supplementation in rheumatoid arthritis patients given very large doses of fish oils administered under reportedly double-blind conditions gave mildly encouraging results. How blinded these studies could be, given the distinctive taste of fish oil, is unclear. Only absence of taste and smell in each patient on such high doses of fish oils could assure blindedness.

An occasional patient with palindromic rheumatism may have an allergic synovitis, but this is quite rare. The impact of diet composition on bacterial gut flora and its importance to reactive arthritis remains an area in need of further research of only theoretical interest at this time. Of more likelihood and concern in the patients we care for are the ability of foodstuffs to modify absorption of medications (e.g., D-penicillamine) and the levels of certain intermediate metabolites (like serum uric acid and plasma lipids).

SUMMARY

In summary, none of the dietary "cures" for rheumatoid arthritis have been well studied or studied in detail, and it is unlikely that any of them will become a panacea. So long as a patient feels his or her diet is tolerable, and you do not think it is so extreme that it is at high risk for producing dietary imbalance, if the patient thinks it "works," leave it alone. However, do remind your patients that "natural" does not equal safe or better. The number of natural poisons and toxic contaminants in edible plants and animals are in the hundreds, so *it is neither safe nor natural* to take *pharmacologic amounts of any substances* that have not been evaluated for safety, let alone efficacy. Do remember, however, that the reason patients look to unorthodox therapies for relief of rheumatic diseases is better proof of the limitations of our treatment than of some innate character fault that makes them prey to charlatans.

SUGGESTED READINGS

1. Ziff M. Diet in the treatment of rheumatoid arthritis. Arthritis Rheum. 1983; 26;457-61.

2. Kremer JM, Jubiz W, Rynes RI, et al. Fish-oil fatty acid supplementation in active rheumatoid arthritis: A double-blinded, controlled cross-over study. Ann Intern Med. 1987; 106: 497-503.

3. Panush RS. Nutritional therapy for rheumatic diseases. Ann Intern Med. 1987; 106:619-21.

INDEX

Page numbers in *italics* denote figures; those followed by "t" denote tables.